Equine Oncology

Editor

ANNA R. HOLLIS

VETERINARY CLINICS OF NORTH AMERICA: EQUINE PRACTICE

www.vetequine.theclinics.com

Consulting Editor
RAMIRO E. TORIBIO

December 2024 • Volume 40 • Number 3

ELSEVIER

1600 John F. Kennedy Boulevard • Suite 1800 • Philadelphia, Pennsylvania, 19103-2899

http://www.vetequine.theclinics.com

VETERINARY CLINICS OF NORTH AMERICA: EQUINE PRACTICE Volume 40, Number 3
December 2024 ISSN 0749-0739, ISBN-13: 978-0-443-12937-7

Editor: Taylor Hayes
Developmental Editor: Akshay Samson

Veterinary Clinics of North America: Equine Practice (ISSN 0749-0739) is published in April, August, and December by Elsevier Inc., 360 Park Avenue South, New York, NY 10010-1710. Business and Editorial Offices: 1600 John F. Kennedy Blvd., Suite 1800, Philadelphia, PA 19103-2899. Subscription prices are $314.00 per year (domestic individuals), $100.00 per year (domestic students/residents), $358.00 per year (Canadian individuals), $391.00 per year (international individuals), $100.00 per year (Canadian students/residents), and $180.00 per year (international students/residents). For institutional access pricing please contact Customer Service via the contact information below. To receive student/resident rate, orders must be accompanied by name of affiliated institution, date of term, and the signature of program/residency coordinator on institution letterhead. Orders will be billed at individual rate until proof of status is received. Foreign air speed delivery is included in all *Clinics* subscription prices. All prices are subject to change without notice. Orders, claims, and journal inquiries: Please visit our Support Hub page https://service.elsevier.com for assistance.

Reprints. For copies of 100 or more of articles in this publication, please contact the Commercial Reprints Department, Elsevier Inc., 360 Park Avenue South, New York, NY 10010-1710. Tel.: 212-633-3874; Fax: 212-633-3820; E-mail: reprints@elsevier.com.

Veterinary Clinics of North America: Equine Practice is covered in *MEDLINE/PubMed (Index Medicus), Excerpta Medica, Current Contents/Agriculture, Biology and Environmental Sciences, and ISI.*

Contributors

CONSULTING EDITOR

RAMIRO E. TORIBIO, DVM, MS, PhD
Diplomate, American College of Veterinary Internal Medicine; Professor and Trueman Endowed Chair of Equine Medicine and Surgery, College of Veterinary Medicine, The Ohio State University, Columbus, Ohio, USA

EDITOR

ANNA R. HOLLIS, BVetMed, MSc (Clin Onc), SFHEA, FRCVS
Diplomate, American College of Veterinary Internal Medicine (Large Animal); Diplomate, European College of Equine Internal Medicine; Teaching Professor, Department of Veterinary Medicine, University of Cambridge, Cambridge, United Kingdom

AUTHORS

JILL BRYAN, BSc (Hons), MVB, FRCPath, MRCVS
Diplomate of the European College of Equine Internal Medicine; Equine Veterinary Pathologist and Medicine Specialist, Irish Equine Centre, Johnstown, Naas, Co. Kildare, Ireland

TERESA A. BURNS, DVM, PhD
Diplomate of the American College of Veterinary Internal Medicine (Large Animal Internal Medicine); Associate Professor, Department of Veterinary Clinical Sciences, College of Veterinary Medicine, The Ohio State University, Columbus, Ohio, USA

PADRAIC M. DIXON, MVB, PhD, FRCVS
Diplomate Equine Veterinary Dental College (Equine); Edinburgh, United Kingdom

CONSTANZE FINTL, BVSc, MSc, PhD
Diplomate European College of Equine Internal Medicine; Senior Lecturer in Equine Medicine, Department of Companion Animal Clinical Sciences, Faculty of Veterinary Medicine and Biosciences, Norwegian University of Life Sciences, Ås, Norway

ANDY FISKE-JACKSON, BVSc, MVetMed, FHEA, MRCVS
Diplomate of the European College of Veterinary Surgeons; Associate Professor of Equine Surgery, Equine Referral Hospital, Royal Veterinary College, Hatfield, Hertfordshire, United Kingdom

ERIC GREEN, DVM
Professor, Department of Veterinary Clinical Sciences, The Ohio State University, The Ohio State University Veterinary Medical Center, Columbus, Ohio, USA

ANNA R. HOLLIS, BVetMed, MSc (Clin Onc), SFHEA, FRCVS
Diplomate, American College of Veterinary Internal Medicine (Large Animal); Diplomate, European College of Equine Internal Medicine; Teaching Professor, Department of Veterinary Medicine, University of Cambridge, Cambridge, United Kingdom

PHILIP IVENS, MA, VetMB, Cert EM (Int Med), MRCVS
Diploma of the European College of Internal Medicine; EBVS European Veterinary Specialist in Equine Internal Medicine, RCVS Specialist in Equine Medicine (Internal Medicine), Managing Director, Buckingham Equine Vets Ltd, Sparrow Lodge Farm, Wicken, Milton Keynes, United Kingdom

IMOGEN JOHNS, BVSc, PGCAP, FRCVS
Diplomate of the American College of Veterinary Internal Medicine; Equine Medicine Specialist, B and W Equine Hospital, Breadstone, Berkeley, Gloucestershire, United Kingdom

FERNANDO MALALANA, DVM, PhD, FHEA, FRCVS
Diplomate of the European College of Equine Internal Medicine; Senior Lecturer in Equine Internal Medicine, Philip Leverhulme Equine Hospital, University of Liverpool, Neston, United Kingdom

INA MERSICH, Mag med vet
Equine Internal Medicine Resident, Department of Veterinary Clinical Medicine, University of Illinois, Urbana, Illinois, USA

MARGARET C. MUDGE, VMD
Clinical Professor of Equine Emergency and Critical Care and Surgery, Department of Veterinary Clinical Sciences, The Ohio State University, The Ohio State University Veterinary Medical Center, Columbus, Ohio, USA

SUZANNE MURPHY, BVM&S, MSc, MRCVS
Diplomate of the European College of Veterinary Internal Medicine-Companion Animals(Oncology); Director of Clinics, Royal (Dick) School of Veterinary Studies University of Edinburgh Easter Bush, United Kingdom

JAMIE PRUTTON, BSc (Hons), BVSc, MBA, CMgr, MCMI, MRCVS
Diplomate of the American College of Veterinary Internal Medicine; Diplomate of the European College of Equine Internal Medicine; RCVS and European Specialist in Equine Internal Medicine, Equine Internal Medicine, Liphook Equine Hospital, Liphook, Hampshire, United Kingdom

AMANDA SAMUELS, VMD, PhD
Equine Internal Medicine Resident, Department of Veterinary Clinical Sciences, College of Veterinary Medicine, The Ohio State University, Columbus, Ohio, USA

VICTORIA SOUTH, MA, VetMB, CertAVP (EM), MRCVS
Diploma of the European College of Internal Medicine; EBVS European Veterinary Specialist in Equine Internal Medicine, RCVS Specialist in Equine Medicine (Internal Medicine), Clinical Lead in Equine Internal Medicine, Department of Veterinary Medicine, University of Cambridge, Cambridge, United Kingdom

RACHEL TUCKER, BSc, BVetMed, MVetMed, CertAVP(ESO), MRCVS
Diplomate of the European College of Veterinary Surgeons; RCVS and European Specialist in Equine Surgery, Equine Surgery, Liphook Equine Hospital, Liphook, Hampshire, United Kingdom

PAMELA A. WILKINS, DVM, MS, PhD
Diplomate of the American College of Veterinary Internal Medicine-LA; Diplomate of the American College of Veterinary Emergency and Critical Care; Professor of Equine Internal Medicine, Department of Veterinary Clinical Medicine, College of Veterinary Medicine, University of Illinois at Urbana-Champaign, Urbana, Illinois, USA

Contents

Cancer is disease of the genome. The Hallmarks of cancer are a way of thinking of cancer to help rationalize what occurs in this disease process. A solid tumor is a complex of normal and neoplastic cells, arising through an evolutionary process to survive and grow. By understanding how normal cellular mechanisms are subverted to promote cancer we can refine our approach to improve outcomes. It gives us opportunities to prevent some cancers and allowing earlier diagnosis. We can refine conventional diagnostic tools and give more accurate prognoses. It offers novel targets to improve treatment of cancers, allowing personalized medicine.

The diagnosis of neoplasia in the horse is both simple and extremely challenging, depending on the type of neoplasm and its location. Obtaining an accurate diagnosis of a neoplastic condition is key to formulating an appropriate treatment plan if possible or developing a palliative plan if curative treatment options do not exist. A combination of historical features, clinical examination findings, and diagnostic testing typically allow a working diagnosis of neoplasia to be made, with a definitive diagnosis requiring the identification of neoplastic cells in a sample or tissue.

Equine neoplasia poses challenges in surgical management owing to their diverse locations and potential for aggressive behavior. Surgical interventions aim for complete excision while minimizing cosmetic and functional impairments. Techniques such as laser ablation and electrochemotherapy offer minimally invasive options for accessible tumors. For deeper or larger masses, surgical excision with adequate margins remains the gold standard. Preoperative biopsy and imaging guides surgical planning, ensuring complete tumor removal while preserving vital structures. Close adherence to a strict surgical protocol to prevent seeding of tumor cells, and, where possible, appropriate skin reconstruction techniques will improve cosmesis and outcome.

Thoracic neoplasia often presents with generalized and nonspecific clinical signs and should be considered as a differential especially when patients are nonresponsive to therapeutic intervention for more common differential diagnoses of respiratory disease (such as equine asthma) and where there is evidence thoracic and/or abdominal effusion upon examination. Antemortem diagnosis can be challenging and working closely with a pathologist to differentiate the respective neoplasia is helpful. Early recognition and appropriate management of thoracic neoplasia are vital for patient welfare as rapid disease progression can be relatively quick, and/or the relatively advanced stage of disease in which these patients frequently present.

There are a number of unusual tumors in the horse. Gross tumor characteristics, anatomical location, and signalment may assist with identification. Clinical pathology is often unrewarding with non-specific findings, while fine needle aspirates may not obtain sufficient tissue material to confirm a diagnosis. Although regular staining of biopsy material may be sufficient, immunohistochemistry markers may be required, especially in less differentiated tumors. The prognosis is dependent on the type, location, tumor size as well as on metastatic spread. A selection of unusual and rare tumors that the clinician is more likely to encounter is discussed.

This article discusses the reported paraneoplastic syndromes (PNSs) in horses, including the possible pathogenesis, diagnostic methods, and any treatment options. The more commonly reported PNSs in horses include cancer anorexia and cachexia, fever and increased acute phase protein concentrations, and hypercalcemia and monoclonal gammopathy. As these conditions can often be more commonly diagnosed in non-neoplastic conditions, the diagnosis of a PNS and the accompanying neoplasia can be challenging. As signs of a PNS may precede signs of the underlying neoplasia, it is important that the clinician be aware of the possible presence of a PNS.

VETERINARY CLINICS OF NORTH AMERICA: EQUINE PRACTICE

SERIES OF RELATED INTEREST

Veterinary Clinics of North America: Food Animal Practice
https://www.vetfood.theclinics.com/

THE CLINICS ARE NOW AVAILABLE ONLINE!
Access your subscription at:
www.theclinics.com

Preface

Equine Oncology: Why Does It Matter Anyway?

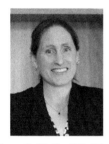

Anna R. Hollis, BVetMed,
MSc (Clin Onc), SFHEA,
FRCVS
Editor

Whilst I would be the first to admit that oncology is not generally considered to be the most important field within equine medicine, this underserved area is growing in understanding, and the treatment options are often varied and complex with very little evidence behind many of the traditional approaches. New treatments are being investigated all the time, and as owners demand better treatment options for their horses, practitioners need to be at the forefront of these developments to best advise the management of these sometimes-complicated cases.

In order to truly move forward in the field of equine oncology, one needs a good understanding of the causes of neoplasia, as well as the principles of management. This issue therefore aims to improve the practitioner's knowledge of equine oncology as a discipline, spanning pathogenesis, treatments, and the latest knowledge of a variety of tumor types and locations. No text on equine oncology can be comprehensive, because our knowledge and understanding are increasing all the time. This issue therefore contains the most relevant areas that the practitioner will benefit from based on the current state of knowledge in the area.

The issue starts with a review of the principles of tumor biology, followed by an overview of the diagnosis and staging of equine neoplasia, in order to equip the practitioner with the skills to work up these cases to the best possible level. Articles focused on the most common treatment options follow to enable the equine practitioner to confidently guide the best treatment of tumors in general. Details of the current knowledge of the pathogenesis and treatment of the most common types of tumors and those found in various areas of the body follow, including the more commonly diagnosed "unusual" tumors. Finally, an article on paraneoplastic syndromes covers how to recognize and manage those syndromes caused by the indirect presence of tumors in the horse.

Vet Clin Equine 40 (2024) xiii–xiv
https://doi.org/10.1016/j.cveq.2024.08.001
0749-0739/24/© 2024 Published by Elsevier Inc.

vetequine.theclinics.com

I would like to thank Dr Ramiro E. Toribio for the invitation to edit and contribute to this issue, and I would especially like to thank the authors, who are all experts in their topics, for their time and generosity in producing their articles to help to advance this subspeciality. This has truly been a labor of love for all concerned, and I am delighted to present this special Equine Oncology issue of *Veterinary Clinics of North America: Equine Practice*. I am confident that this issue will become a valuable resource for equine practitioners and the aspiring equine practitioners of the future, and I hope that readers enjoy it as much as I have.

Anna R. Hollis, BVetMed, MSc (Clin Onc), SFHEA, FRCVS
Department of Veterinary Medicine
University of Cambridge
Madingley Road
Cambridge CB3 0ES, UK

E-mail address:
arh207@cam.ac.uk

Principles of Tumor Biology

Suzanne Murphy, BVM&S, MSc, MRCVS

KEYWORDS

- Equine • Neoplasia • Molecular

KEY POINTS

- Cancer is a disease of the genome.
- Molecular aberrations arise allowing cells to reproduce without the influence of mechanisms that control the number and integrity of normal cells.
- These aberrations may occur randomly, be inherited, or caused through infectious or environmental carcinogens.
- Cancer cells can manipulate the tumor microenvironment, subverting normal mechanisms to provide an environment in which the tumor can flourish.
- Understanding the molecular basis of cancer gives further opportunities to prevent, diagnose, prognosticate, and treat it more successfully.

INTRODUCTION

The word "cancer" like the word "infection," is a broad term. It is used to describe a pathologic process involving uncontrolled cell growth and proliferation. There are about 200 different cancers with different behaviors and outcomes. Cancer, like an infection, can be rapidly devastating and fatal, or curable and minor depending on the tumor type involved.

It can be described as a disease of the genome, with a cancer arising from the accumulation of several genetic mutations that act in a way that eliminates normal regulation of cell proliferation and impacts on genetic integrity. This in turn allows the proto-cancer cells to acquire other mutations that are needed for a cancer to develop and survive within the body.

The initial mutations can either be inherited or acquired as part of the inherent error rate of accurately replicating each of the approximately 2.7 billion base pairs in a horse's DNA during normal cell division. They can be driven by other mutagens (environmental or infectious) which directly or indirectly increase the rates of repair of DNA within the target tissue, and thus increase the risk of errors.

When a mutation arises the impact it has depends on the effect it has on the protein coded for. They can be irrelevant—being either silent, meaning that the cell continues to function normally, or they can be fatal to the cell, so the cell fails to replicate and

Royal (Dick) School of Veterinary Studies, University of Edinburgh, Easter Bush, EH25 9RG, UK
E-mail address: Sue.murphy@ed.ac.uk

Vet Clin Equine 40 (2024) 341–350
https://doi.org/10.1016/j.cveq.2024.07.001
0749-0739/24/© 2024 Elsevier Inc. All rights reserved, including that for text and data mining, AI training, and similar technologies.

pass on the mutation. However, some mutations provide a step along the pathway to that cell's progeny becoming neoplastic. The genes that are involved in maintaining DNA integrity from cell cycle to cell cycle are particularly important. Once these gate-keepers cease to function properly each cell's daughter cells are inherently genetically unstable, and will express more genetic mutations, some of which will confer a survival advantage to that particular cell line and ultimately give rise to the initial clonal expansion of 1 cell that categorizes the development of a tumor.

There are an estimated 22,000 protein coding genes in the horse that can be randomly switched "on" or "off" as part of this genetic instability to confer that survival advantage. The easiest way to consider this in more detail is to look at the "hallmarks of cancer."

HALLMARKS OF CANCER

In 2000 Douglas Hanahan and Robert Weinberg proposed that cancer could be defined through six "hallmarks…. that could be used as an organizing principle for rationalizing the complexities of neoplastic disease."[1] This proposal was updated in 2011 to include 2 further hallmarks and 2 "enablers" that promoted cancer development.[2]

The 8 hallmarks are reproduced in **Box 1**.

The hallmarks can be further categorized into those associated with cell cycle dysregulation and aberrant cancer cell metabolism and those associated with manipulation of the non-neoplastic cells within the body to produce an environment supporting the development of the cancer.

Cell Cycle Dysregulation

The drive to undergo mitosis is driven by growth factors, and their presence or absence. It is regulated to maintain the right number of cells—a "cellular homeostasis." In cancer, the neoplastic cell ignores growth factors or growth inhibitors.

A common example of this is the disruption of receptor tyrosine kinase signaling pathways in many neoplastic cells. In normal mammalian cells, there are specific transmembranous receptor tyrosine kinases which can be thought of as "on" and "off" switches for cell proliferation. They are switched "on" by growth promoting factors interacting with the extra-cellular receptor of the tyrosine kinase, which allows

---

Box 1
Hallmarks of cancer

- Self-sufficiency in growth signals,
- Insensitivity to growth-inhibitory (antigrowth) signals
- Evasion of programmed cell death (apoptosis)
- Limitless replicative potential
- Sustained angiogenesis (ability to produce new blood supply to supply oxygen and nutrients to the tumor)
- Tissue invasion and metastasis
- Dysregulation of metabolic pathways
- Evasion of the immune system

phosphorylation of the intracellular component of the receptor and leads to a cascade of intracellular events resulting in cell division. No growth factor present means no phosphorylation and thus no proliferation. There have been 58 receptor tyrosine kinases identified in humans. Their dysregulation is important in the development of human cancers and happens in different ways including gain-of-function mutations whereby the phosphorylation occurs in the absence of growth factor.[3]

An example where well-documented mutations allow the intracellular domain of the receptor kinase to be phosphorylated perpetually is found in canine mast cell tumors. KIT (CD117) is a receptor tyrosine kinase found on mast cells and has been found to be mutated in such a way in about 15% to 35% of canine mast cell tumors.[4]

An aberrance in KIT expression (no mutation was looked for) has been identified in an oral mast cell tumor in the horse[5] and it is known that the Bovine papilloma virus (BPV) oncoprotein E5 binds to another receptor tyrosine kinase, in this case platelet-derived growth factor β receptor, causing phosphorylation and activation in equine fibroblasts that ultimately contributes downstream toward the development of a sarcoid.[6]

Telomerase and cell cycle dysregulation

A normal differentiated cell has a limited number of times it can reproduce itself after which the cell becomes senescent. This is referred to as the Hayflick limit. The number is thought to vary from cell type to cell type and is regulated by the length of the chromosomal telomeres. The telomeres are a repetitive sequence of DNA that are on the end of each chromosome to protect the chromosome from becoming tangled or stuck to other chromosomes during replication. Telomeres decrease in length after every cell division and eventually cease to be present, at which point the cell stops being able to reproduce successfully.[7] An enzyme called telomerase is present in gametes, stem cells, and some other cell types, and acts to restore the diminished telomeres, allowing the Hayflick limit to be surpassed. Therefore by "switching on" telomerase cancers can have a *limitless reproductive potential*. It also provides an opportunity for the development of anti-telomerase treatments to treat cancer.

Cell reproduction is one side of the equation. Programmed cell death (apoptosis) is also an important part of cell number homeostasis. Unlike necrosis, which results from a traumatic acute cellular injury, apoptosis is highly regulated and controlled within the body. Therefore any mechanism that renders a cell immune to this process contributes to cancer formation.

A well-known apoptotic pathway involves *p53*. *P53* was one of the earliest identified tumor suppressor genes, sometimes referred to as the "guardian of the genome." During mitosis its function is to promote apoptosis in any daughter cells with aberrant, unrepairable DNA variance from the original cell. Inactivation of p53 through its mutation therefore removes an important regulator of genetic stability.

Dysregulation of metabolic pathways

Cancer cells are often in a hypoxic environment, and for the cells to survive and flourish a rearrangement of metabolic pathways occurs so that the cells can thrive regardless of the levels of oxygen surrounding them.

These cells have increased glucose uptake and increased lactate production, regardless of oxygen levels, whereas normal cells take up glucose and convert it to lactate only in the absence of oxygen.[8] This is called the "Warburg effect" after the man who discovered it in the 1920s.

Recently there has been interest in when this phenomenon occurs-is it 'before, as a result of, or in combination with, the genetic changes driving cancer.[9]' It has also been appreciated that there are metabolic pathways other than the glucose pathway that are altered in cancer cells , involving amino acid metabolism and lipid metabolism.

Extracellular Effects of Cancer Cells

For cancer cells to thrive they must interact with normal cells, subverting them into creating a pro-cancer microenvironment. The hallmarks of cancer referring to tissue invasion and metastasis, sustained angiogenesis, and evasion of the immune system describe this.

Malignant tumors have the capacity to invade local structures and metastasise. Metastasis is the major reason cancers kill. Metastasis is a multistep process, which is captured in **Box 2**. This ability is driven by the acquisition of a genetic profile by the cancer cell that allows it to switch on or off genes within the cell, allowing these steps to occur.

As an aside, it should be noted that benign lesions grow in an expansile manner. However, these lesions still have the capacity to induce clinical problems due to their space occupying nature (eg, intracranial meningiomas) or can be considered otherwise "malignant by location" such as pedunculated intra-abdominal lipomas which can cause entrapment and torsion of the intestine in older horses.

Angiogenesis is a term describing the process of new blood vessel formation and occurs in embryologic development, tissue repair, and reproductive processes. It is also necessary for solid tumor growth. As a cancer develops beyond about 2 mm in size, areas furthest away from existing blood vessels become hypoxic. Neoplastic cells stimulate the formation of new blood vessels by releasing various growth factors. A key growth factor family is the vascular endothelial growth factor family. These growth factors promote the proliferation and migration of normal non-neoplastic endothelial cells to form new blood vessels to provide oxygen and nutrients to allow the mass to grow.[10]

Transformation of cells into neoplastic cells is thought to happen in the body all the time. However, one of the reasons cancers do not get established as a consequence, is due to immunosurveillance. The immune system can *eliminate* an early cancer, allow *equilibrium* with the cancer, thus resulting in the tumor being dormant, or the cancer can *escape* the influence of the immune system—the "three E's theory."[11]

The tumor can "escape" through several mechanisms. For example, tumors can downregulate the expression of major histocompatibility complex (MHC) class 1 molecules. MHC I molecules are found on all cells. Their role is to present peptides from the proteins synthesized by those cells. In healthy cells, all these proteins are ones to which CD8+ T cells are tolerant, so recognized as "self." However, when cells are expressing mutant sequences "non-self" peptides are presented, allowing the immune system to detect and destroy these cells. If there is down regulation, the tumor cell is not recognized as abnormal and so not removed.[12] This is known to occur in

---

Box 2
Steps in metastasis

For a cancer to undergo metastasis there needs to be
- Local *invasion*
- *Intravasation* into blood vessels (or invasion into lymphatics)
- *Survival* within the blood/lymphatics
- The ability to *adhere* to the vessel wall in the target organ
- And then *extravasation* into that new location and the setting up of a microenvironment conducive to survival there.

equine sarcoid development where BPV E5 down regulates MHC I transcription in equine fibroblasts.[13]

Neoplastic cells can also release various factors that inhibit the activity of the immune system and the hypoxic, hypoglycaemic, acidic, amino acid depleted tumor microenvironment can further inhibit the immune response. Additionally, T regulatory cells (T reg) are often increased in the tumor locale, their presence mediated by the cancer cells. T reg cells dampen the immune response and are important in stopping an excessive or abnormal immune response in a normal animal. Their increase has the effect again of protecting the cancer from the immune system.[14]

Inflammation and Cancer

In the update to their original hallmarks of cancer paper, 10 years later Hanahan and Weinberg named inflammation, together with genomic instability, as "enablers of cancer."[2]

Inflammation is not only important as part of the host immune response, but is also important in repair and remodeling of tissue after trauma. However, inflammation also has a role in cancer initiation and progression, not only dampening the immune response to cancer cells, but also creating a pro-cancer microenvironment. It is argued that the mechanisms necessary for normal tissue growth and repair are the same mechanisms utilized for cancer growth, which then end up in a positive feedback loop whereby the inflammation caused by the presence of the tumor promotes the continued existence of the tumor. It is thought that infection, chronic inflammation, or autoimmune interactions at the same tissue or organ site precedes cancer in about 20% of all human cancers[15] Chronic inflammation associated squamous cell carcinoma (SCC) has been seen in horses with previous eye injuries, after burns or other injury, associated with long-standing conjunctivitis, and with eyelid deformities.[16]

CANCER AS A MICROSCOPIC ECOSYSTEM

Sometimes it seems like a cancer has agency, developing strategies that allow it to thrive. In reality the development of cancer is more like the Darwinian model of evolution, with the genetically unstable cell producing progeny that have random genetic mutations, some of which confer a survival advantage, some of which are fatal, some of which are dead ends.

A solid tumor therefore is a complex ecosystem, made up of heterogeneous subpopulations of tumor cells with different genotypes and therapeutic susceptibilities.[17] The tumor cells are intermingled with non–neoplastic cells recruited by the cancer to promote growth and metastasis (such as endothelial cells that form the blood vessels), or to help escape the immune system (eg, Treg cells). Alternatively, the non–neoplastic cells can be part of the healthy immune response to the cancer such as cytotoxic T cells. Areas of the tumor will be necrotic, hypoxic, inflamed, and the tumor cells more or less differentiated. Cells will be multiplying at different rates. All of this will change over different time points as neoplastic clones proliferate, die out and influence the tumor microenvironment. To add more complexity, it is also thought that cancer cells can switch behavior in response to environmental stresses and therapeutic pressure without genomic alterations, referred to as cell plasticity.[18]

Thus, any one moment in time a mass may be composed of many neoplastic cells, all with a fundamentally similar but differing genetic profile, together with some normal macrophages, fibroblasts, lymphocytes and blood vessels hijacked into producing the ideal microenvironment for the tumor to survive in at that moment in its evolution. Sampling the same tumor hours or days later would identify subtle differences both within the neoplastic cells, the normal cells and the soup of cytokines within the mass, as the environmental pressures such as hypoxia, pH and diffusion gradients impact on the survival advantage of different tumor clones.

This heterogenous nature is one of the reasons that tissue sampling to reach a diagnosis can be challenging, where sometimes a needle biopsy may miss sampling the identifiable tumor cells but sample associated inflammation or necrosis instead. Even bigger incisional biopsies can miss the more representative areas of the tumor, leading to an underestimation of the grade or even a misdiagnosis.

CAUSES OF CANCER

Cancer can be considered to arise broadly from heritable, environmental or infectious causes, and there is frequently an interplay between multiple factors to cause it.

Although most cancer arises from random mutations that occur as part of normal cell turnover in the body, there are also individuals born with mutations in the germline (therefore in all cells in the body) that increase the risk of developing a particular cancer, which may also be passed on to their offspring. A good example of a single gene having such an effect is the 'breast cancer' gene (*BRCA1*) in humans. This gene produces a protein important in DNA repair. Individuals inheriting a mutation in *BRCA1* have a 72% chance of developing breast cancer before the age of 80 years old. In comparison, people without the mutation have a 13% chance.[19] Everyone inherits two copies of the *BRCA1* gene. In any individual, there is a chance that a mutation will occur in *BRCA1* as a random event. Once both wild type *BRCA1* alleles have been mutated in a particular cell the tumor suppressing effect of this gene is lost and that cell is one step closer to being transformed into a neoplastic cell. This is referred to as Knudson's two hit hypothesis-you need 'two hits' to knock out both alleles.[20] In an individual born with one mutated gene in every cell, it is more likely that the second copy will be mutated in the same cell somewhere along the line, as a random event. This explains why cancer tends to arise earlier in those carrying a germline mutation, and often in multiple sites.

It can be argued that breeds of animals are analogous to human families, inheriting susceptibility to different types of cancer. This is recognized in dogs, where it is mostly thought to be the influence of many genes with low penetrance acting in concert to increase the risk of certain cancer types, but less clear in horses. We do know that certain breeds where there is a high incidence of gray horses there is also a high risk of melanoma associated with those horses. The gray gene is an autosomal dominant one, with horses homozygous or heterozygous for the gene becoming gray as they age. This is the most common reason for horses to be white, and seems to originate from an ancient common ancestor.[21] Greying seems to be driven by a mutation in STX17 modified by the expression or otherwise of several other genes which gives rise to four different clinical traits. The *STX17* mutation is the major contributor, and the other genes have individually a small but significant effect when summated. Horses homozygous for the greying gene have a higher risk of developing melanoma and at a younger age.[22]

Environmental and infectious agents are also associated with an increased risk of developing cancer. In humans there are well known environmental drivers associated with cancer, with arguably the most well-known being cigarette smoke. There are also different occupations and areas of the world that are associated with increased risks of developing different sorts of cancer. For example, exposure to ionizing radiation, asbestos and heavy metals as well as eating certain foodstuffs are associated with increased risks of developing different types of tumors. Infectious causes of cancer include human papilloma virus (HPV), Human Immunodeficiency virus (HIV) and

Helicobacter pylori in humans. It can be many years before the cancer becomes evident after the exposure to the carcinogen making the identification of carcinogens sometimes challenging.

Ultraviolet light is a known carcinogen associated with the development of SCC of certain anatomic sites in species such as humans, cattle, and cats. As with other species, SCC in the horse is likely of multifactorial origin. Tumors associated with chronic ultraviolet light damage are seen on the head of lightly colored horses with an increased incidence of this tumor being associated with geographic areas of high altitude or with long hours of sunshine.[23] Hair acts as a barrier to UV damage so these SCC arise on sparsely haired or hairless non-pigmented areas. Commonly they are periocular or involving the globe or orbit. SCC of the vulva has also been seen in depigmented skin at the mucocutaneous junction.[24] As the whole depigmented area is exposed to the carcinogen, it is possible to see several lesions in the same area exhibiting different stages of development from actinic pre-cancerous change through carcinoma—in -situ to more advanced SCC.

There is also a published case series of horses with ocular and periocular hemangiosarcoma and a case report of a vulval hemangiosarcoma with associated solar elastosis, suggesting a UV light etiopathology in these cases.[25,26]

There is compelling evidence for viral involvement in the development of certain equine cancers. BPVs have been known to be involved in the development of equine sarcoids for nearly 90 years and more recently, equine papilloma viruses have been implicated in the development of equine genital SCC.[27] Equus caballus papillomavirus 2 sequences have been identified in genital and ocular SCC[28] as well as stomach and nasal and oral SCC,[29] whereas BPV 1, 2, and 13 have been implicated in the development of sarcoids.[29] The papilloma genome can be divided into early (E) and late (L) coding regions based on the time of viral protein expression during infection. Some of the early and, more recently, the late coding regions have been identified as contributing to tumor development.

RELEVANCE TO THE CLINICIAN
Prevention

By understanding the mechanisms by which cancer arises, we can decrease the incidence of some cancers by developing breeding strategies that minimize the risks. We can try to avoid events that increase the risk of mutagenesis, for example, keeping lightly pigmented horses out of the midday sun, or vaccinate against infectious causes of cancer. There are now human papilloma virus vaccines, to prevent cervical cancer, and work ongoing looking at the role vaccination might have in preventing sarcoids.

Diagnosis

We can refine conventional methods of diagnosis by looking for gene expression associated with particular cancers and improve the accuracy of prognosis by looking for certain molecular signatures associated with a good or, conversely, a poor outcome. These techniques can increasingly be carried out using liquid biopsies— such as blood, cerebrospinal fluid (CSF), ascitic fluid, and urine. Looking for cell-free DNA; circulating tumor cell DNA or circulating tumor cells in these liquids can allow diagnosis of hard to biopsy lesions, identify cancer residual disease after treatment or spot recurrence earlier, increasing options for early intervention in a relatively non-invasive way.[30] We can use the existence of genetic profiles known to be associated with certain types of cancer to diagnose and screen for that cancer to catch it earlier in the course of the disease.

Treatment

Traditional cancer therapies such as surgery, radiotherapy, and conventional chemotherapy are relatively insensitive tools, destroying normal tissues as well as neoplastic ones and relying on repair mechanisms of the normal tissue to reverse the adverse effects of the treatment. Often the toxicity of the treatment is the limiting factor for dose escalation, so the therapeutic index is small, and side effects relatively common. Radiotherapy and chemotherapy are in themselves mutagenic, and thus carcinogenic.

By gaining greater understanding of what is happening at a molecular level, novel treatment modalities can be developed that exploit the differences between normal and neoplastic tissues. We can design molecules to target the disease process while sparing normal cells. We can identify what is happening in an individual's tumor and decide whether a particular treatment would be of benefit. As we understand the tumor's microenvironment and how it supports the cancer, we can manipulate it to be less supportive. These targeted therapies are likely to compliment the existing therapeutic options that are available.

There is frequent overlap of strategies. For example, overexpression of COX-2 in different types of carcinomas in humans and domestic animals is associated with an increased survival of neoplastic cells. Its expression is pro-angiogenic, invasive, and metastatic in many cancers.

In humans, large clinical studies using long-term non-steroidal anti-inflammatories have shown a decreased incidence in some cancer types for people taking these drugs. In dogs established treatment for urothelial cell cancer of the bladder (transitional cell carcinoma) includes COX-2 inhibitors. The investigation of expression of COX-2 using immunohistochemistry in equine SCC and melanoma has given varied results.[31] There is a report of use of piroxicam for at least 6 months in a mare after a revision cystoplasty for a SCC of the apex of the bladder with no recurrence.[32] There is another report of using piroxicam to control an SCC of the lip with success.[31]

There has been a revival of the use of immunotherapy in recent years with some exciting successes in reversing the mechanisms by which tumors escape the immune system. There are different strategies with different targets and different outcomes, depending on how the tumor of interest evades the immune system.

A DNA vaccine used in the treatment of canine oral malignant melanoma has been used for the last nearly 20 years. It targets tyrosinase, which is a glycoprotein uniquely essential in the development of melanocytes. The technology involves injecting a plasmid vector coding for a xenogeneic tyrosinase to cause cross-reactivity and trigger an autoimmune response. Any side effects therefore are limited to melanin-producing cells or from administering a foreign protein. The vaccine has been used in horses off licence for over 10 years with one recent review suggesting some clinical benefit.[33]

There is an increasing use of immune check point inhibitors in human medicine which act to stop the normal immune check point process, which is in itself modified by tumor escape mechanisms. The inhibition of the immune check point process is not without its risks of immune-related side effects to normal tissues and the understanding and utilization of these treatments is being refined.[34]

SUMMARY

The complete sequencing of the human genome, followed by that of the dog and then the horse[35] together with the technological and digital revolution that allows rapid gene sequencing, and analysis of gene expression now allows us an understanding of cancer a magnitude greater than ever before. There is a golden opportunity to make a bigger impact in prevention and treatment of this group of diseases, including the horse. Equine oncology is very much in its infancy as a science in comparison to human, but the fundamentals of mammalian cell biology are the same from species to species and the same opportunities broadly apply.

CLINICS CARE POINTS

- It is important to sample any suspect lesion knowing that solid tumors often have areas of necrosis and inflammation, which may give unrepresentative results.
- Tumors have different behaviors depending on their cell of origin.
- The grade of a tumor is the aggressiveness of a tumor within its histologic type.
- Once the diagnosis is made a thorough clinical examination helps identify the stage of the disease. Knowing the tumor type and its likely behavior helps to focus the examination.
- Palpation is a poor indicator of lymph node metastasis. Cytology is more reliable.
- Knowing stage and grade helps with both prognostication and treatment plan.

DISCLOSURE

There are no affiliations other than I (S. Murphy) work for the University of Edinburgh.

REFERENCES

1. Hanahan D, Weinberg RA. The hallmarks of cancer. Cell 2000;100(1):57–70.
2. Hanahan D, Weinberg RA. Hallmarks of cancer: the next generation. Cell 2011; 144(5):646–74.
3. Du Z, Lovly CM. Mechanisms of receptor tyrosine kinase activation in cancer. Mol Cancer 2018;17:58.
4. Blackwood L, Murphy S, Buracco P, et al. European consensus document on mast cell tumours in dogs and cats. Vet Comp Oncol 2012;10(3):1–29.
5. Seeliger F, Heß O, Pröbsting M, et al. Confocal laser scanning analysis of an equine oral mast cell tumor with atypical expression of tyrosine kinase receptor C-KIT. Veterinary Pathology 2007;44(2):225–8.
6. Ogłuszka M, Starzyński RR, Pierzchała M, et al. Equine sarcoids—causes, molecular changes, and clinicopathologic features: a review. Veterinary Pathology 2021;58(3):472–82.
7. Deng Y, Chan S, Chang S. Telomere dysfunction and tumour suppression: the senescence connection. Nat Rev Cancer 2008;8:450–8.
8. Koppenol WH, Bounds PL, Dang CV. Otto Warburg's contributions to current concepts of cancer metabolism. Nat Rev Cancer 2011;11(5):325–37. Erratum in: Nat Rev Cancer. 2011 ;11(8):618. PMID: 21508971.
9. Hirschey MD, DeBerardinis RJ, Diehl AME, et al. Target Validation Team. Dysregulated metabolism contributes to oncogenesis. Semin Cancer Biol 2015; 35(Suppl):S129–50.
10. Pérez-Gutiérrez L, Ferrara N. Biology and therapeutic targeting of vascular endothelial growth factor A. Nat Rev Mol Cell Biol 2023;24:816–34.
11. Fridman Wolf H. From cancer immune surveillance to cancer immunoediting: birth of modern immuno-oncology. J Immunol 2018;201(3):825–6.
12. Rock KL, Reits E, Neefjes J. Present Yourself! By MHC Class I and MHC Class II Molecules. Trends Immunol 2016;37(11):724–37.

13. Marchetti B, Gault EA, Cortese MS, et al. Bovine papillomavirus type 1 oncoprotein E5 inhibits equine MHC class I and interacts with equine MHC I heavy chain. J Gen Virol 2009;90(Pt 12):2865–70.

14. Ohue Y, Nishikawa H. Regulatory T (Treg) cells in cancer: Can Treg cells be a new therapeutic target? Cancer Sci 2019;110(7):2080–9.

15. Greten FR, Grivennikov SI. Inflammation and cancer: triggers, mechanisms, and consequences. Immunity 2019 16;51(1):27–41.

16. Knottenbelt DC, Croft JS. Cutaneous squamous cell carcinoma (SCC): "What's the problem?". Equine Vet Educ 2019;31:635–46.

17. Zahir N, Sun R, Gallahan D, et al. Characterizing the ecological and evolutionary dynamics of cancer. Nat Genet 2020;52:759–67.

18. Vendramin R, Litchfield K, Swanton C. Cancer evolution: Darwin and beyond. EMBO J 2021 15;40(18):e108389.

19. Kuchenbaecker KB, Hopper JL, Barner DR, et al. Risks of breast, ovarian, and contralateral breast cancer for BRCA1 and BRCA2 mutation carriers. JAMA 2017;317(23):2402–16.

20. Chernoff J. The two-hit theory hits 50. Mol Biol Cell 2021;32(22):rt1.

21. Pielberg G, Golovko A, Sundström E, et al. A cis-acting regulatory mutation causes premature hair graying and susceptibility to melanoma in the horse. Nat Genet 2008;40(8):1004–9.

22. Tesena P, Kingkaw A, Vongsangnak W, et al. A preliminary study: proteomic profiling uncovers potential proteins for biomonitoring equine melanocytic neoplasm. Animals (Basel) 2021;11(7):1913.

23. Dugan SJ, Curtis CR, Roberts SM, et al. Epidemiologic study of ocular/adnexal squamous cell carcinoma in horses. J Am Vet Med Assoc 1991;198:251–325.

24. Raś A, Otrocka-Domagała I, Raś-Noryńska M. Two different clinical forms of squamous cell carcinoma (SCC) in the perineum and vulva of two mares. BMC Vet Res 2020;16:464.

25. Scherrer NM, Lassaline M, Engiles J. Ocular and periocular hemangiosarcoma in six horses. Vet Ophthalmol 2018;21(4):432–7.

26. Gumber S, Baia P, Wakamatsu N. Vulvar epithelioid hemangiosarcoma with solar elastosis in a mare. J Vet Diagn Invest 2011;23(5):1033–6.

27. Nasir L, Brand S. Papillomavirus associated diseases of the horse. Vet Microbiol 2013;167:159–67, 1–2.

28. Jones SE. Papillomaviruses in equids: A decade of discovery and more to come? Equine Vet Educ 2022;34:236–40.

29. Miglinci L, Reicher P, Nell B, et al. Detection of equine papillomaviruses and gamma-herpesviruses in equine squamous cell carcinoma. Pathogens 2023;12(2):179.

30. Nikanjam M, Kato S, Kurzrock R. Liquid biopsy: current technology and clinical applications. J Hematol Oncol 2022;15(1):131.

31. Smith KM, Scase TJ, Miller JL, et al. Expression of cyclooxygenase-2 by equine ocular and adnexal squamous cell carcinomas. Vet Ophthalmol 2008;11(Suppl 1):8–14.

32. Serena A, Naranjo C, Kock C, et al. Resection cystoplasty of a squamous cell carcinoma in a mare. Equine Vet Educ 2009;21:263–6.

33. Pellin MA. The use of oncept melanoma vaccine in veterinary patients: a review of the literature. Vet Sci 2022;9(11):597.

34. Esfahani K, Roudaia L, Buhlaiga N, et al. A review of cancer immunotherapy: from the past, to the present, to the future. Curr Oncol 2020;27(Suppl 2):S87–97.

35. Brosnahan MM, Brooks SA, Antczak DF. Equine clinical genomics: A clinician's primer. Equine Vet J 2010;42(7):658–70.

Diagnosis and Staging of Equine Neoplasia

Imogen Johns, BVSc, FRCVS[a],*, Jill Bryan, MVB, FRCPath, MRCVS[b]

KEYWORDS

- Neoplasia • Diagnosis • Biopsy • Cytology • Staging

KEY POINTS

- Diagnosis of equine neoplasia typically requires a combination of diagnostic modalities.
- Confirmation of the type of tumor is made via cytologic/histopathologic examination of specimens.
- Staging is used to help plan appropriate treatment and better understand prognosis.

INTRODUCTION

The diagnosis of neoplasia in the horse is both simple and extremely challenging, depending on the type of neoplasm and its location. A small, pigmented nodule around the anus of a middle-aged gray horse is highly likely to be a melanoma, and further diagnostics are rarely necessary. Gradual weight loss and intermittent dullness in an older gelding could be caused by a myriad of conditions, ranging from dentition issues to endocrine disorders to neoplasia. In general, external neoplastic conditions that can be seen or palpated externally tend to be easier to diagnose than internal neoplasia, because at least in some cases the lesion appearance is close to pathognomonic but also because sampling of a lesion to obtain a definitive diagnosis is considerably easier. In horses with internal neoplasia, a stepwise, logical approach to the investigation of clinical signs, with appropriate ancillary diagnostics including ultrasound, radiography, and in some cases more advanced imaging techniques, can lead to a working diagnosis of neoplasia. This article discusses how a working diagnosis of neoplasia is made using clinical signs and a range of diagnostic tools, and how it is confirmed using cytologic or histopathologic techniques.

HOW DOES NEOPLASIA RESULT IN CLINICAL DISEASE?

The presence of neoplasia, in particular internal (ie, that which cannot be seen externally) neoplasia, can result in clinical signs via several different processes. First is the

[a] B and W Equine Hospital, Breadstone, Berkeley GL67QD, UK; [b] Irish Equine Centre, Johnstown, Naas, Co. Kildare, Ireland
* Corresponding author.
E-mail address: imogen.johns@bwequinevets.co.uk

Vet Clin Equine 40 (2024) 351–369
https://doi.org/10.1016/j.cveq.2024.07.002
0749-0739/24/© 2024 Elsevier Inc. All rights reserved, including those for text and data mining, AI training, and similar technologies.
vetequine.theclinics.com

so-called mass effect, where the size of the neoplastic mass itself causes clinical signs. For example, a pulmonary granular cell tumor (GCTs) within the tracheal lumen is likely to be clinically silent until it reaches a size whereby airflow is impeded and respiratory stridor and distress develop.[1] Second, the neoplastic cells can interfere with the normal function of an organ resulting in clinical signs. Infiltrative intestinal lymphoma results in weight loss (and other signs) caused predominately by a malabsorptive process secondary to neoplastic cell infiltration into the intestinal wall.[2] Third, the tumor may produce substances that result in clinical signs distant to the tumor itself, a so-called paraneoplastic syndrome. Finally, although seemingly rare in horses, metastatic lesions may result in clinical signs at sites distant to the primary tumor.

CLINICAL SIGNS IN HORSES WITH EXTERNAL NEOPLASIA

The most common cutaneous tumors in horses are sarcoids, melanomas, and squamous cell carcinomas.[3] Clinical signs can vary from none at all in small tumors at sites that do not interfere with function to significant ulceration/bleeding of lesions causing pain and discomfort and mass effect especially with large melanomas around the anus, which can impact passage of feces resulting in colic and discomfort (**Fig. 1**).

Diagnosis of External Neoplasia

Clinical appearance of lesions forms the basis for the diagnosis of external neoplasia, but should always be confirmed with histopathology to ensure an accurate diagnosis is made.

In one study of equine sarcoids, relying on the clinical appearance of the lesions for diagnosis was shown to have an overall sensitivity of 83.3% and specificity of 79.6%.[4]

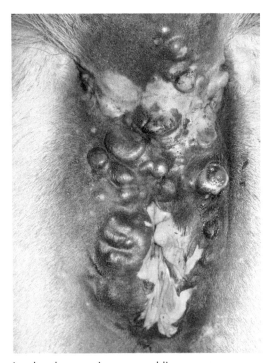

Fig. 1. Multiple perianal melanomas in a gray gelding.

In an associated study, the same authors developed and validated a diagnostic protocol, which used age of the animal, history of tumor growth, number and anatomic location of lesions and lesion morphology.[5] Using an online examination whereby respondents did or did not use the diagnostic protocol, overall the odds for respondents who did use the diagnostic protocol (DP) to correctly diagnose a case were 1.2 times higher than those not using it (odds ratio, 1.25; 95% confidence interval, 1.09–1.43), an effect that was greater in clinicians with less than 1 year experience (odds ratio, 1.58; 95% confidence interval, 1.13–2.19) suggesting that this may be a useful tool to aid in the diagnosis of equine sarcoids.

The most common external locations for squamous cell carcinomas are penile/preputial and ocular. The gross appearance can vary significantly between horses and various anatomic sites, and can be either proliferative or erosive (and in some cases both).[6] Local tissue invasion can cause significant tissue necrosis and associated signs. Similar to sarcoids, a definitive diagnosis of lesion type can only be made following histopathologic assessment of a lesion. In particular for penile/preputial lesions, palpation/ultrasound to detect lymphadenopathy and possibly sampling (biopsy or fine-needle aspirates [FNA]) of local lymph nodes is important to determine the possibility of local spread. Metastasis was confirmed in 14/82 (17.1%) horses in one study.[7]

CLINICAL SIGNS IN HORSES WITH INTERNAL NEOPLASIA

Tumors affecting the thoracic and abdominal cavities typically cause nonspecific signs of disease including weight loss, anorexia, and intermittent fevers.[1,2,8,9] Primary pulmonary tumors are uncommon in horses; however, GCTs are the most frequently reported primary lung tumor with lymphoma being the most common hematopoietic tumor affecting the thoracic cavity.[1] Signs relating to thoracic cavity involvement may include cough, respiratory distress, ventral edema, and epistaxis.[1,10] Within the thoracic cavity, primary and metastatic tumors can affect the pulmonary parenchyma, the pleural cavity, the mediastinum, and associated lymph nodes, and the predominant clinical signs may vary depending on where the lesions are located. For example, when a tumor causes compression of the airway (either externally or internally) then coughing and increased respiratory effort/distress is typically more pronounced, whereas in cases with (often large volume) pleural effusion, dyspnea is more commonly noted, with ventral edema especially with mediastinal involvement. A rare occurrence in some horses with thoracic tumors is the development of hypertrophic osteopathy[11] (Marie disease), a paraneoplastic syndrome resulting in periosteal proliferation of new bone and soft tissue swelling along diaphyses of long bones. The swelling is painful and horses often have a shuffling gait.

In two case series of 68 horses with intestinal neoplasia, the most common historical signs included weight loss, colic (acute onset and intermittent), anorexia, fever, depression, diarrhea, and ventral edema.[2,9] Similar signs were noted in 24 horses with gastric neoplasia, although hypersalivation was also noted in 7/24.[8] Primary tumors affecting abdominal organs are rare and include renal carcinoma,[12] hepatoblastoma, hepatocellular carcinoma,[13] and hemangiosarcoma,[14] with clinical signs typically nonspecific.

Tumors of the male reproductive tract (apart from squamous cell carcinoma) are uncommon, with seminomas being the most frequently reported. These typically result in rapid enlargement of the testicle and can metastasize.[6,15] In mares, GCTs are benign tumors of the ovaries that can result in clinical signs because of abnormal hormonal activity or related to a mass effect. Stallion-like behavior is a commonly reported behavioral sign in mares with GCT, and in a recent retrospective study was found to be significantly associated with increased concentrations of testosterone, antimüllerian hormone (AMH), inhibins, and inhibin-B.[16] In the same study, there was no increase in any of these hormone concentrations in mares with other behavioral changes including aggression, suggesting that these clinical signs cannot be attributed to a GCT. Uterine tumors are rare and are typically benign with leiomyoma being most common. Clinical signs may not be apparent if the mare is not used for breeding. If clinical signs are present, infertility can occur, and uterine hemorrhage may also be noted.[17]

Diagnosis of Internal Neoplasia

Because the clinical signs of internal neoplasia are typically nonspecific, additional diagnostic testing is typically required. The choice of tests depends on the presenting signs of the animal, the suspected body system affected, and the availability of diagnostic modalities, and can include the following:

1. Clinical examination
2. Routine hematology and biochemistry
3. Potential biomarkers
4. Ultrasonography
5. Radiography
6. Endoscopy
7. Computed tomography
8. MRI
9. Laparoscopy and thoracoscopy
10. Cytology
11. Tissue biopsy

CLINICAL EXAMINATION

Along with obtaining a full history, a full clinical examination is an essential first step. Identification of external masses/lesions, palpation for possible lymphadenopathy, and evidence of signs, such as ventral edema, may all help with guiding the most appropriate next diagnostic step. In horses with abdominal pain or weight loss, a rectal palpation should also be part of the clinical examination.

Routine Hematology and Biochemistry

There are no pathognomonic findings on routine clinical pathology that allow confirmation of a diagnosis of neoplasia. Nonspecific findings in horses with internal neoplasia can include anemia, hyperproteinemia and hypoproteinemia, and increased levels of acute phase proteins, although these can also be seen in many nonneoplastic disorders.[2,9]

Potential Tumor Biomarkers

Various tumor biomarkers have been shown to be useful in the diagnosis of neoplasia in humans and small animals. Studies in horses are limited, although it is an area of ongoing research and some more recently investigated biomarkers are discussed next. Based on current knowledge, it is recommended that the measurement of a relevant tumor biomarker should only be performed in horses that have clinical or laboratory findings of the suspected disease, rather than being used as a general screening test.[18]

Thymidine Kinase

Thymidine kinase (TK) is a cellular enzyme involved in DNA synthesis and increased serum TK activity has been associated with neoplastic disease in humans, in particular hematologic neoplasia.[19–21] Increased serum TK activity has also been associated with lymphoma in dogs and cats[22,23] and in dogs it has been shown to have prognostic value.[24] Some studies performed in horses have shown that higher serum TK activity is helpful in differentiating horses with lymphoma from those with inflammatory disease and nonhematopoietic neoplasia, although there was some overlap between these groups and sensitivity of the test was low.[25,26] However, other studies have showed no association between serum TK1 activity and lymphoma in horses.[27] Overall, based on current knowledge, measurement of serum TK activity can sometimes be a useful adjunct test in cases of suspected lymphoma, with high serum TK activity increasing the index of suspicion of lymphoma; however, lymphoma cannot be ruled out in horses with low serum TK activity and the accuracy of the methods of measurement requires further investigation.

Antimüllerian Hormone

Endocrinologic panels including measurement of inhibin, testosterone, and progesterone have been used to aid in the diagnosis of GCTs in mares. More recently, AMH produced by granulosa cells has been shown to be a clinically useful biomarker for the diagnosis of GCTs in mares.[28–30] Serum AMH concentrations are considered more sensitive than inhibin, testosterone, or the combination of inhibin and testosterone for detection of GCTs in mares and AMH also has the advantage of not being significantly affected by pregnancy or the stage of the estrus cycle.[30]

MicroRNAs

MicroRNAs are recognized biomarkers in humans for various diseases, including certain types of neoplasia, where they may also have prognostic value and are considered potential future therapeutic targets.[31–33] In horses, microRNAs have been proposed as potential biomarkers for equine sarcoids and although more research is needed, there is some potential that microRNAs may represent potential diagnostic and prognostic biomarkers, such as potentially being able to help identify horses at higher risk of sarcoid development.[34–36]

Ultrasonography

Ultrasonography is a useful diagnostic tool to identify and characterize internal and external abnormalities.[37] Percutaneous ultrasound of the abdomen and thorax should follow a systematic approach with the aim of identifying abnormalities, such as masses, increase in size of an organ, thickening of intestinal walls, increased volumes of peritoneal and pleural fluid, and abnormal echogenicity of organs.[38,39] Rectal ultrasound is used in horses in which a palpable abnormality was detected per rectum, and can also be used to assess for possible tumors of the mare reproductive tract. Because of the large size of the equine abdomen, the entire abdomen cannot be imaged. Despite this, abnormal findings on ultrasound are commonly reported in horses with intestinal and thoracic neoplasia (**Figs. 2 – 4**).[8,9,40] In one case series, 21/23 horses that had abdominal ultrasound performed had abnormalities identified including thickening of intestinal walls and identification of a mass.[9] Ultrasonographic findings in horses with thoracic neoplasia can include increased volume of pleural fluid (often very large volume and anechoic in appearance[41]), pleural surface irregularities

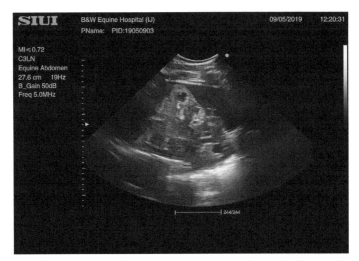

Fig. 2. Large multiloculated neoplastic mass with associated pleural effusion. The mass was visible in multiple intercostal spaces and the cranial mediastinum. [With permission from SIUI (Shantou Institute of Ultrasonic Instruments Co., Ltd.).]

including parenchymal masses, masses within the pleural cavity, and masses/fluid within the cranial mediastinum.[1] Masses that are surrounded by normally aerated lung tissue cannot be seen via ultrasound, but may be visible radiographically, depending on their size and location.[1]

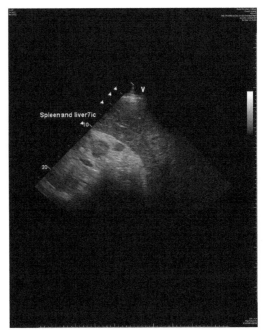

Fig. 3. Ultrasonographic image of an aged gray gelding with weight loss. Multiple masses of varying echogenicity were visible within the splenic parenchyma.

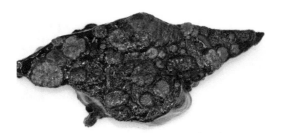

Fig. 4. Spleen of horse in **Fig. 3** showing multiple nodules throughout parenchyma. These were confirmed as melanoma.

Radiography

The large size of the mature equine abdomen precludes the utility of radiography as a diagnostic aid in horses with suspected abdominal neoplasia. Thoracic radiographs are used to diagnose primary and metastatic pulmonary neoplasia. If pleural effusion is present, this should be drained before radiographs being taken because lesions may be obscured by the fluid. Focal opacities are seen with solitary GCTs, whereas more numerous diffuse opacities are seen with metastatic disease. Obtaining bilateral radiographs may increase the sensitivity of radiographs. In a recent study, a pulmonary mass would have been missed in one of seven horses if only one side of the thorax was radiographed.[42] Radiographs of suspected neoplastic lesions of other areas in the body, such as distal limbs and head, may show evidence of bony proliferation or lysis/destruction, or pressure atrophy secondary to adjacent soft tissue masses (**Fig. 5**).[43,44]

Endoscopy

Endoscopy is used to directly visualize tumors within the nasal cavity including paranasal sinuses, respiratory tract, urogenital tract, and gastrointestinal tract.[1,7,9,45–47] Direct visualization may also allow for obtaining a biopsy for histopathologic analysis, although samples are typically small and may not always be diagnostic because of associated inflammation and necrosis in parts of the tumor. Gastroscopy with biopsy is the diagnostic tool of choice for diagnosis of gastric neoplasia (**Fig. 6**). Every effort should be made to search for metastases, because in one case series, 18/23 horses had metastatic disease.[7]

Computed Tomography

The increased availability of standing computed tomography (CT) of the head has greatly advanced the ability to diagnose and implement appropriate treatment of neoplastic conditions of the head.[44,48–51] CT allows for cross-sectional imaging and multiplanar reconstruction providing a greater ability to assess the extent of a lesion, to determine the presence of surrounding tissue involvement and if appropriate, to allow detailed presurgical planning to be performed (**Fig. 7**). In some cases differentiation of tumor tissue from surrounding normal tissue is challenging because they may have a similar tissue density and thus attenuation on CT images. In these cases, intravenous contrast is used to highlight the tumor, which typically has alterations of blood flow compared with normal tissue.[50] Because of the need for exact timing of the CT after contrast injection, this is best performed under general anesthesia. CT evaluation of the limb can also be used to further investigate suspected neoplastic conditions, although at present, the large size of the adult horse precludes imaging of other sites, such as the abdomen or thoracic cavity.[52]

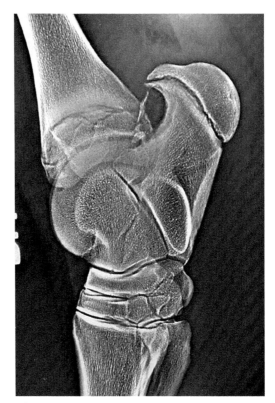

Fig. 5. Radiograph of a young horse with multiple masses of the distal limbs, showing a smooth-bordered radiotranslucent defect. Hemangiosarcoma was diagnosed.

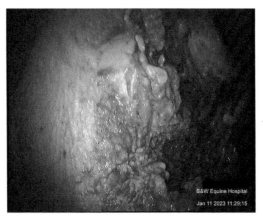

Fig. 6. Large invasive mass in the stomach. Suspected gastric squamous cell carcinoma. (Courtesy image by B&W Equine Hospital.)

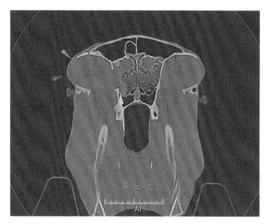

Fig. 7. CT image from horse with unilateral exophthalmos (*blue and orange arrowheads*) and blindness. The CT showed a soft tissue attenuating tissue associated with the optic cone extending to infiltrate the ethmoturbinates (*yellow arrow*). Although a biopsy was not obtained, the mass was suspected to be neoplastic.

MRI

MRI is considered superior to CT for evaluation of soft tissue structures.[52] In contrast to distal limb MRI, which is performed in the standing sedated horse, MRI of the head requires a prolonged general anesthesia and its availability is limited. Neoplastic conditions were diagnosed in a group of 84 horses undergoing head MRI in one study, with good correlation between imaging and surgical/postmortem findings.[53]

Laparoscopy and Thoracoscopy

Laparoscopy and thoracoscopy can allow for direct visualization of a suspected tumor. Biopsy samples may then be taken allowing for a definitive diagnosis, or in some cases, most commonly mares with ovarian GCTs, removal of the neoplastic organ can occur. For horses with suspected intrathoracic neoplasia, ultrasound-guided percutaneous biopsy is used to sample focal masses, although this is typically used for the diagnosis of more diffuse lung disease.[54] Thoracoscopy is typically well tolerated in the standing sedated horse, even those with advanced lung disease, and allows access to and direct visualization of the dorsal and dorsolateral aspects of the lung. Biopsy samples are obtained from visualized masses or enlarged lymph nodes.[55–59]

Laparoscopy is performed in the standing or recumbent horse. Depending on the area of interest, the left flank and right flank approaches in the standing horse and the ventral approach in the dorsally recumbent horse is used.[60] Laparoscopy was performed in 3/34 horses in one series and 2/34 horses in a second series of horses with intestinal neoplasia allowing for antemortem diagnosis in these horses.[2,9]

CONFIRMING THE DIAGNOSIS

Once a working diagnosis of neoplasia has been made, confirmation of the diagnosis and the type of tumor requires identification of neoplastic cells in samples obtained for cytologic or histopathologic examination.

Cytology

Collection of samples for cytologic examination is a minimally invasive and usually simple technique that is cost effective and allows for rapid diagnostic assessment.

Samples suitable for cytologic examination include FNAs taken directly from masses within the skin, subcutis, internal organs, or body cavities, impression smears, fluid aspirated from body cavities (peritoneal fluid, pleural fluid, pericardial fluid), tracheal wash and bronchoalveolar lavage fluid, synovial fluid, and cerebrospinal fluid.

Cytologic assessment can sometimes be a valuable tool in the diagnosis of certain types of equine tumors, leading to a definitive diagnosis, or if not definitively diagnostic it can sometimes be helpful to distinguish between neoplastic and nonneoplastic lesions or narrow the list of clinical differentials. However, some common equine tumors exfoliate cells poorly on FNA or within body cavities leading to nondiagnostic samples being more common in equine cases as compared with small animals and there is not always agreement between cytologic findings and final histopathologic diagnosis.[61] In one study of 10 horses with histologically confirmed abdominal neoplasia, neoplasia was diagnosed in five of these cases based on cytologic examination of peritoneal fluid, with a definitive diagnosis reached in four horses,[62] whereas in another study 11 out of 25 horses with abdominal neoplasia had an accurate diagnosis based on cytologic examination of peritoneal fluid, although repeated examination was sometimes required.[63] Types of neoplasms that exfoliate cells more easily on FNA or within body cavities and therefore may be more easily diagnosed on cytology include lymphoma, melanomas, and mast cell tumors, whereas equine sarcoids and other types of mesenchymal tumors often exfoliate cells poorly, even on FNA (**Figs. 8** and **9**). Given its limited sensitivity, it is important to remember that the absence of neoplastic cells on cytologic examination often does not completely exclude the possibility of a neoplastic lesion and tissue biopsy may be required for further investigation.

Tissue Biopsy

Tissue biopsy for histopathologic examination is often the most helpful diagnostic test in investigating cases of suspected neoplasia because in many cases it leads to an accurate diagnosis, or at least narrows down a list of possible differential diagnoses. Although more invasive than an FNA, biopsy samples from various types of lesions can often be obtained in the standing horse and histologic examination of tissue has the advantage of allowing assessment not only of cell types present but also tissue architecture and how neoplastic cells are interacting with normal tissues and it more commonly leads to a definitive diagnosis (**Fig. 10**).

There are concerns that taking biopsy samples from certain types of neoplasms may exacerbate the lesion and overall clinical progression. Reports in the literature

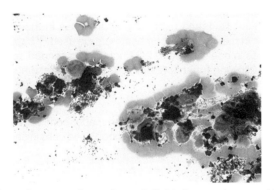

Fig. 8. Neoplastic melanocytes in peritoneal fluid from a horse with an abdominal melanoma.

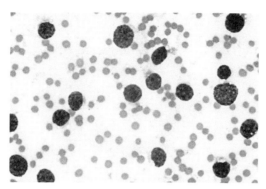

Fig. 9. Neoplastic lymphocytes in pleural fluid from a horse with mediastinal lymphoma.

are lacking; however, there have been frequent anecdotal reports of this occurring following incisional biopsies of sarcoids, although it is difficult to predict how an individual neoplasm will respond. When taking biopsies from these lesions it is preferable to perform excisional biopsies if possible or to have a treatment plan in place that can be implemented as soon as the histopathologic diagnosis is received.

How to Take a Good Biopsy Sample in Cases of Suspected Neoplasia

For diagnostic investigation in cases of suspected neoplasia the aim is to collect a representative tissue sample for histopathologic examination. An excisional biopsy (complete removal of the lesion) or incisional biopsy (removal of a portion of the lesion) can be performed and factors influencing the type of biopsy to obtain include the size of the lesion, accessibility of the lesion, equipment available, ability/experience of the clinician, and the suspected diagnosis.

Excisional biopsies

Submission of an excisional biopsy of a lesion and surrounding tissue has the advantage of allowing the pathologist to assess neoplastic cells in all areas of the lesion and assessing how neoplastic cells are interacting with normal tissue, which can increase the likelihood of reaching a definitive diagnosis (**Fig. 11**). It also allows for potential treatment of the lesion at the same time as diagnosis and allows for assessment of

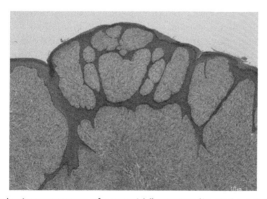

Fig. 10. Histopathologic appearance of a sarcoid (hematoxylin-eosin, original magnification 20×).

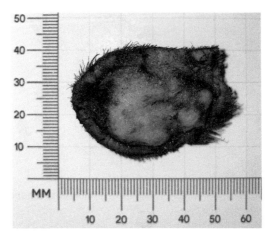

Fig. 11. Excisional biopsy of a cutaneous mass.

surgical margins, which can help to determine if additional treatment might be required. Despite these advantages, excisional biopsies are not always possible to obtain and are more readily achieved with cutaneous lesions that are often of a smaller size.

Incisional biopsies

In some cases, it is challenging to clinically differentiate neoplastic and nonneoplastic lesions (eg, chronic inflammatory lesions) or to clinically differentiate between different types of neoplasms. Incisional biopsies are therefore sometimes preferred to try to reach a diagnosis before planning surgical and/or medical treatment and are also appropriate for lesions in which an excisional biopsy cannot be readily obtained (eg, because of lesion size or location). Types of incisional biopsies include punch biopsies, wedge biopsies, Tru-Cut biopsies, and endoscopic biopsies and selection of the most appropriate method of biopsy depends on the suspected diagnosis, location of the lesion (eg, cutaneous/subcutaneous vs in a body cavity/internal organ), and the depth of the lesion (eg, depth within skin/subcutis). When considering the most appropriate type of biopsy sample, it is useful to consider what areas of the lesion are likely to be most representative based on the differential diagnoses.

- Punch biopsies are easy to obtain and minimally invasive and are appropriate for some superficial skin tumors that often extend to the epidermal junction (eg, squamous cell carcinomas, sarcoids, melanomas); however, their small size and superficial nature means they can miss lesions deeper in the dermis and may not always be fully representative of the entire lesion (**Figs. 12** and **13**). Superficial tissue may also be complicated by secondary inflammatory changes (eg, ulceration and granulation tissue) that may conceal other underlying pathology.
- Incisional wedge biopsies generally allow for histopathologic examination of larger areas of tissue than punch biopsies, including areas of the neoplasm and ideally also regions in which neoplastic cells interact with normal tissue.
- Tru-Cut biopsies only sample small areas of tissue but are helpful when suspected neoplasms are within body cavities or internal organs, or are located deeper within subcutaneous tissue or muscle (**Fig. 14**).
- Endoscopic biopsies only allow for sampling of very small superficial areas of tissue but is helpful when larger tissue samples cannot be readily obtained (eg, suspected neoplasia affecting the proximal gastrointestinal tract, investigation of

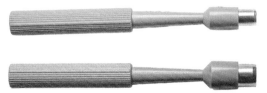

Fig. 12. Punch biopsy instruments.

lesions within the pharynx or guttural pouch) (**Fig. 15**). Their superficial nature is problematic for achieving diagnosis of lesions that are deeper in the submucosa.

Use of a combination of biopsy types (eg, punch biopsies for superficial areas and Tru-Cut biopsies for deeper areas of a large mass) is sometimes beneficial to ensure representative samples are being obtained. Submitting biopsy samples from multiple areas of a lesion should also be considered, and is helpful in increasing the certainty of a histopathologic diagnosis in some cases, such as taking incisional biopsies from the center of a lesion and from the periphery of a lesion where interaction between neoplastic cells and normal tissue can be assessed.

How to Get the Most from Your Biopsy Sample

To ensure you get the most from your biopsy sample it is important to handle the tissue carefully to avoid crush artifact interfering with histopathologic interpretation. For optimal cell preservation tissue should be immediately placed into an appropriate volume of fixative (usually 10% neutral buffered formalin, with a 1:10 tissue to formalin ratio considered ideal). Samples should be submitted to the laboratory in a leak-proof container that allows for easy removal of the sample once it is fixed.

If assessment of surgical margins is required, try to avoid slicing into the sample before fixation, or if a sample is very large only cut into it away from the areas of the margins to allow for additional formalin penetration of tissue. Submitting appropriate clinical information along with the biopsy sample is essential to allow for the most accurate interpretation of the histopathologic findings by the pathologist.

Immunohistochemistry

Immunohistochemical staining of tissue biopsy sections can sometimes be helpful for pathologists when a definitive type of neoplasm cannot be determined from

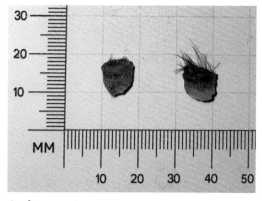

Fig. 13. Punch biopsies from a cutaneous mass.

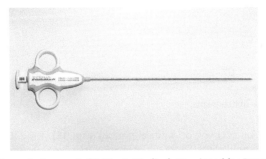

Fig. 14. Tru-Cut biopsy instrument. (© Merit Medical, Reprinted by Permission.)

examination of routine histologic sections alone, or it may at least be helpful to narrow the list of differential diagnoses; however, the range of available antibodies validated in equine tissue is limited compared with what is available for human and small animal samples.

Staging and Grading

Although treatment options may be limited for some if not many neoplastic conditions in horses, if treatment is to be considered, staging is recommended because this may help guide appropriate treatment and prognosis.[64] The TNM system is widely used in human oncology and can be applied to equine tumors, although to date there are limited publications that specifically use a staging system (**Table 1**). Assessment for local and distant metastatic lesions is generally performed by palpation of local lymph nodes and by using appropriate imaging techniques, as previously described. Because of the size of the mature horse and the associated limitations in imaging the thorax and abdomen and accessing lymph nodes, assessment for metastatic spread is challenging, which makes staging difficult in some cases. If local lymph nodes are palpably enlarged and are accessible, FNAs and/or biopsies for cytologic and/or histopathologic examination could be performed to try to detect metastatic lesions; however, because metastatic neoplastic cells are often multifocal within a lymph node, the absence of neoplastic cells on an FNA or incisional biopsy cannot completely exclude the possibility of metastasis. Also, if the tumor or surrounding tissue is inflamed, local lymph nodes may be enlarged as a result of inflammation, rather than metastatic spread of the tumor.

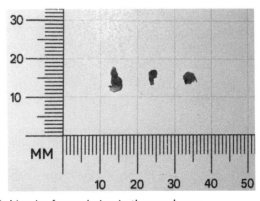

Fig. 15. Endoscopic biopsies from a lesion in the esophagus.

Table 1
The TNM system commonly used in human oncology to assist with staging of disease

T (tumor)	Tumor size and possible invasion of adjacent structures
N (lymph node)	Are any local or draining lymph nodes affected?
M (metastasis)	Are there distant metastases?

Grading of a tumor requires histopathologic examination of a biopsy sample and can provide information on the predicated biologic behavior of a tumor, which is helpful in determining prognosis and in guiding clinical decision making. In small animals there are some well-established grading systems for certain tumor types (eg, canine mast cell tumors, canine soft tissue sarcomas)[65–67]; however, well-validated systems for equine tumors are lacking. A grading system using histopathologic features related to degree of differentiation has been used for squamous cell carcinoma of the equine penis with correlation shown between lower grades (well-differentiated tumors) and a lower rate of metastases; however, further validation of this system is required.[68]

SUMMARY

The approach to the diagnosis of neoplasia in the horse relies on using all available and appropriate diagnostic tools, but should always start with a thorough history and clinical examination. With the advent of advanced imaging modalities, additional diagnostic testing is now available, although the sheer size of the horse still precludes some of the more commonly performed testing in small animals and humans. Obtaining diagnostic samples can also be challenging and invasive considering the size of the horse. Although treatment options may be limited in many cases of internal neoplasia, the increasing interest of owners in obtaining a diagnosis if feasible may then result in additional treatment options becoming available.

CLINICS CARE POINTS

- A diagnosis of neoplasia is based on clinical signs and the results of diagnostic testing and is confirmed by identification of neoplastic cells in sampled tissues/fluids.

- When taking biopsy samples for histopathologic examination, consider what areas of the lesion are likely to be most representative based on the possible differential diagnoses.

- Staging of neoplasia should be attempted because it may help guide appropriate treatment and determine prognosis.

DISCLOSURE

No conflicts of interest of funding declared by either author.

REFERENCES

1. Davis EG, Rush BR. Diagnostic challenges: equine thoracic neoplasia. Equine Vet Educ 2013;25:96–107.
2. Taylor SD, Pusterla N, Vaughan B, et al. Intestinal neoplasia in horses. J Vet Intern Med 2006;20:1429–36.

3. Shaffer PA, Wobeser B, Martin LER, et al. Cutaneous neoplastic lesions of equids in the central United States and Canada: 3,351 biopsy specimens from 3,272 equids (2000–2010). JAVMA 2013;242:99–104.

4. Koch C, Martens A, Hainisch EK, et al. The clinical diagnosis of equine sarcoids - Part 1: Assessment of sensitivity and specificity using a multicentre case-based online examination. Vet J 2018;242:77–82.

5. Haspeslagh M, Gerber V, Knottelnbelt DC, et al. The clinical diagnosis of equine sarcoids – Part 2: assessment of case features typical of equine sarcoids and validation of a diagnostic protocol to guide cequine clinicians in the diagnosis of equine sarcoids. Vet J 2018;240:14–8.

6. Brinsko SP. Neoplasia of the male reproductive tract. Vet Clin N Am Equine Pract 1998;14:517–33.

7. Van den Top JGB, Harkema L, Lange C, et al. Expression of p53,Ki67, EcPV2- and EcPV3 DNA, and viral genes in relation to metastasis and outcome in equine penile and preputial squamous cell carcinoma. Equine Vet J 2014;47:88–195.

8. Taylor SD, Haldorson GJ, Vaughan B, et al. Gastric neoplasia in horses. J Vet Intern Med 2009;23:1097–102.

9. Spanton JA, Smith LJ, Sherlock SE, et al. Intestinal neoplasia: a review of 34 cases. Equine Vet Educ 2020;32:155–65.

10. Mair TS, Brown PJ. Clinical and pathological features of thoracic neoplasia in the horse. Equine Vet J 1993;25:220–3.

11. Mair TS, Tucker RL. Hypertrophic osteopathy (Marie's disease) in horses. Equine Vet Educ 2004;16(6):308–11.

12. Wise LN, Bryan JN, Sellon DC, et al. A retrospective analysis of renal carcinoma in the horse. J Vet Intern Med 2009 Jul-Aug;23(4):913–8.

13. Beeler-Marfisi J, Arroyo L, Caswell J, et al. Equine primary liver tumors: a case series and review of the literature. J Vet Diagn Invest 2010 Mar;22(2):174–83.

14. Southwood LL, Schott HC, Henry CJ, et al. Disseminated hemangiosarcoma in the horse: 35 cases. J Vet Intern Med 2000;14:105–19.

15. Valentine BA. Equine testicular tumours. Equine Vet Educ 2009;21:177–9.

16. Huggins L, Norris J, Conley A, et al. Abnormal mare behaviour is rarely associated with changes in hormonal markers of granulosa cell tumours: a retrospective study. Equine Vet J 2023;56(4):759–67.

17. McCue P. Neoplasia of the female reproductive tract. Vet Clin Nth Am Equine Pract 1998;14:505–15.

18. Drozdzewska K, Gehlen H. Markers for intestinal neoplasia in the horse. Veterinary Medicine and Science 2023;9:32–143.

19. Gronowitz JS, Hagberg H, Källander CF, et al. The use of serum deoxythymidine kinase as a prognostic marker, and in the monitoring of patients with non-Hodgkin's lymphoma. Br J Cancer 1983;47(4):487–95. https://doi.org/10.1038/bjc.1983.78.

20. Hallek M, Wanders L, Strohmeyer S, et al. Thymidine kinase: a tumor marker with prognostic value for non-Hodgkin's lymphoma and a broad range of potential clinical applications. Ann Hematol 1992;65(1):1–5. https://doi.org/10.1007/BF01715117.

21. ZHOU J, HE E, SKOG S. The proliferation marker thymidine kinase 1 in clinical use. Mol Clin Oncol 2013;1(1):18–28. https://doi.org/10.3892/mco.2012.19.

22. von Euler H, Einarsson R, Olsson U, et al. Serum thymidine kinase activity in dogs with malignant lymphoma: a potent marker for prognosis and monitoring the disease. J Vet Intern Med 2004;18(5):696–702. https://doi.org/10.1111/j.1939-1676.2004.tb02608.x.

23. Taylor SS, Dodkin S, Papasouliotis K, et al. Serum thymidine kinase activity in clinically healthy and diseased cats: a potential biomarker for lymphoma. J Feline Med Surg 2013;15(2):142–7. https://doi.org/10.1177/1098612X12463928.

24. Von Euler HP, Rivera P, Aronsson AC, et al. Monitoring therapy in canine malignant lymphoma and leukemia with serum thymidine kinase 1 activity: evaluation of a new, fully automated non-radiometric assay. Int J Oncol 2009;34(2):505–10. https://doi.org/10.3892/ijo_00000175.

25. Larsdotter S, Nostell K, von Euler H. Serum thymidine kinase activity in clinically healthy and diseased horses: a potential marker for lymphoma. Vet J 2015;205(2):313–6. https://doi.org/10.1016/j.tvjl.2015.01.019.

26. Wang L, Unger L, Sharif H, et al. Molecular characterization of equine thymidine kinase 1 and preliminary evaluation of its suitability as a serum biomarker for equine lymphoma. BMC Mol Cell Biol 2021;22(1). https://doi.org/10.1186/s12860-021-00399-x.

27. Moore C, Stefanovski D, Luethy D. Clinical performance of a commercially available thymidine kinase 1 assay for diagnosis of lymphoma in 42 hospitalized horses (2017-2020). J Vet Intern Med 2021;35(5):2495–9. https://doi.org/10.1111/jvim.16239.

28. Almeida J, Ball BA, Conley AJ, et al. Biological and clinical significance of anti-Müllerian hormone determination in blood serum of the mare. Theriogenology 2011;76(8):1393–403.

29. Ball BA, Conley AJ, MacLaughlin DT, et al. Expression of anti-Müllerian hormone (AMH) in equine granulosa-cell tumors and in normal equine ovaries. Theriogenology 2008;70(6):968–77. https://doi.org/10.1016/j.theriogenology.2008.05.059.

30. Ball BA, Almeida J, Conley AJ. Determination of serum anti-Müllerian hormone concentrations for the diagnosis of granulosa-cell tumours in mares. Equine Vet J 2013;45(2):199–203. https://doi.org/10.1111/j.2042-3306.2012.00594.x.

31. Ghafouri-Fard S, Shoorei H, Taheri M. Role of microRNAs in the development, prognosis and therapeutic response of patients with prostate cancer. Gene 2020;759:144995.

32. Iorio MV, Croce CM. MicroRNA dysregulation in cancer: diagnostics, monitoring and therapeutics. A comprehensive review. EMBO Mol Med 2012;4(3):143–59.

33. Piletič K, Kunej T. MicroRNA epigenetic signatures in human disease. Arch Toxicol 2016;90(10):2405–19. https://doi.org/10.1007/s00204-016-1815-7.

34. Unger L, Gerber V, Pacholewska A, et al. MicroRNA fingerprints in serum and whole blood of sarcoid-affected horses as potential non-invasive diagnostic biomarkers. Vet Comp Oncol 2019;17(1):107–17.

35. Cosandey J, Hamza E, Gerber V, et al. Diagnostic and prognostic potential of eight whole blood microRNAs for equine sarcoid disease. PLoS One 2021;16(12 December). https://doi.org/10.1371/journal.pone.0261076.

36. Unger L, Abril C, Gerber V, et al. Diagnostic potential of three serum microRNAs as biomarkers for equine sarcoid disease in horses and donkeys. J Vet Intern Med 2021;35(1):610–9. https://doi.org/10.1111/jvim.16027.

37. Johns IC. Ultrasonography as an aid to the antemortem diagnosis of internal neoplasia in the horse. Equine Vet Educ 2024;36:128–30.

38. Freeman SL. Diagnostic ultrasonography of the mature equine abdomen. Equine Vet Educ 2003;15:319–30.

39. Hillyer MH. The use of ultrasonography in the diagnosis of abdominal tumours in the horse. Equine Vet Educ 1994;6:273–8.

40. Janvier V, Evrard L, Cerri S, et al. Ultrasonographic finings in 13 horses with lymphoma. Vet Radiol Ultrasound 2016;57:65–74.

41. Johns IC, Marr C, Durham A, et al. Causes of pleural effusion in horses resident in the UK. Equine Vet Educ 2017;29:144–8.
42. Malek G, Leclere M, Masseau I, et al. Bilateral thoracic radiographs increase lesion detection in horses with pneumonia or pulmonary neoplasia but do not bring any additional benefit for inflammatory or diffuse pulmonary disease. Vet Radiol Ultrasound 2022;63:518–29.
43. Johns I, Stephen J, Del Peiro F, et al. Hemangiosarcoma in 11 young horses. J Vet Intern Med 2005;19:564–757.
44. Cissell DD, Wisner ER, Textor J, et al. Computed tomographic appearance of equine sinonasal neoplasia. Vet Radiol Ultrasound 2012;53:245–51.
45. Quéré E, Bourzac C, Farfan M, et al. Standing hand-assisted laparoscopic diagnosis and treatment of a rare case of uterine adenocarcinoma in an 18-year-old mare. J Equine Vet Sci 2019 Aug;79:39–44.
46. Dixon PM, Head KW. Equine nasal and paranasal sinus tumours: part 2: a contribution of 28 case reports. Vet J 1999;157:279–94.
47. Dixon PM, Parkin TD, Collins N, et al. Equine paranasal sinus disease: a long-term study of 200 cases (1997-2009)L ancillary diagnostic findings and involvement of the various sinus compartments. Equine Vet J 2012;44:267–71.
48. Tucker R, Windley ZE, Abernethy AD, et al. Radiographic, computed tomographic and surgical anatomy of the equine sphenopalatine sinus in normal and diseased horses. Equine Vet J 2016;48:578–84.
49. Morgan RE, Fiske-Jackson AR, Hellinge M, et al. Equine odontogenic tumours: clinical presentation, CT findings, and outcome in 11 horses. Vet Radiol Ultrasound 2019;60:50–512.
50. Dixon J, Weller R. Advanced diagnostic imaging for neoplastic processes in the head. Equine Vet Educ 2015;27:9–10.
51. Dixon J, Smith K, Perkins J, et al. Computed tomographic appearance of melanomas in the equine head: 13 cases. Vet Radiol Ultrasound 2016;57:246–52.
52. Nagel H, Lang H, Sole Guitart A, et al. Multi-modality imaging of aggressive submural neoplasia of the hoof in two horses. Aust Vet J 2022;100:336–41.
53. Maso-Diaz G, Dyson S, Dennis R, et al. Magnetic resonance imaging characteristics of equine head disorders: 84 cases (2000-2013). Vet Radiol Ultrasound 2015;56:176–87.
54. Venner M, Schmidbauer S, Drommer W, et al. Percutaneous lung biopsy in the horse: comparison of two instruments and repeated biopsy in horses with induced acute intersitial pneumopathy. J Vet Intern Med 2006;20:968–73.
55. Pollock P, Russell T. Standing thoracoscopy in the diagnosis of lymphosarcoma in a horse. Vet Rec 2006;159:354–6.
56. Fry MM, Magdesian KG, Judy CE, et al. Antemortem diagnosis of equine mesothelioma by pleural biopsy. Equine Vet J 2003;35:723–7.
57. Facemire PR, Chilcoat CD, Sojka JE, et al. Treatment of granular cell tumour via complete lung resection in a horse. J Am Vet Med Assoc 2000;217:1522–5.
58. Ford TS, Vaala WE, Sweeney CR, et al. Pleuroscopic diagnosis of gastroesophageal squamous cell carcinoma in a horse. J Am Vet Med Assoc 1987;190:1556–68.
59. Lee WL, Tennent-Brown BS, Barton MH, et al. Two horses with thoracic lymphoma diagnosed using thoracoscopic biopsy. Equine Vet Educ 2013;25:79–83.
60. Martens A, Haart A. Role of laparoscopy in diagnosis and management of equine colic. Vet Clin North Am Equine Prat 2023;39:339–49.
61. Zachar EK, Burgess HJ, Wobeser BK. Article fine-needle aspiration in the diagnosis of equine skin disease and the epidemiology of equine skin cytology

submissions in a Western Canadian diagnostic laboratory. Can Vet J 2016;57(6): 629–34.

62. Recknagel Tierarztpraxis König S, Fritz Schusser G, Recknagel S, et al. Diagnostic assessment of peritoneal fluid cytology in horses with abdominal neoplasia Diagnostische Aussagekraft Der Zytologie von Bauch-Punktaten Bei Abdominalen. Tumoren Des Pferdes 2012. Available at: https://www.researchgate.net/publication/224819638.

63. Zicker SC, Wilson WD, Medearis I. Differentiation between intra-abdominal neoplasms and abscesses in horses, using clinical and laboratory data: 40 cases (1973-1988). J Am Vet Med Assoc 1990;196(7):1130–4. Available at: http://europepmc.org/abstract/MED/2329084.

64. Ensink JM. Why clinicians should consider tumour staging and grading in horses. Equine Vet J 2015;47:141.

65. Kuntz CA, Dernell WS, Powers BE, et al. Prognostic factors for surgical treatment of soft-tissue sarcomas in dogs: 75 cases (1986–1996). J Am Vet Med Assoc 1997;211(9):1147–51. https://doi.org/10.2460/javma.1997.211.09.1147.

66. Avallone G, Rasotto R, Chambers JK, et al. Review of histological grading systems in veterinary medicine. Vet Pathol 2021;58(5):809–28. https://doi.org/10.1177/0300985821999831.

67. Kiupel M, Webster JD, Bailey KL, et al. Proposal of a 2-tier histologic grading system for canine cutaneous mast cell tumors to more accurately predict biological behavior. Vet Pathol 2011;48(1):147–55. https://doi.org/10.1177/0300985810386469.

68. Van den Top JGB, de Heer N, Klein WR, et al. Penile and preputial squamous cell carcinoma in the horse: a retrospective study of treatment of 77 cases. Equine Vet J 2008;40:533–7.

Surgical Management of Equine Neoplasia

Andy Fiske-Jackson, BVSc, MVetMed, DECVS

KEYWORDS

• Equine • Neoplasia • Tumors • Surgery • Margins • Skin reconstruction

KEY POINTS

• Early intervention improves outcomes in patients with cancer.
• The first attempt at excision represents the greatest chance of a successful outcome.
• Neoadjunctive therapy represents an opportunity to improve outcomes.
• Preoperative biopsy will report the appropriate surgical dose.
• Numerous surgical techniques exist to facilitate skin closure following tumor excision.

INTRODUCTION

Equine neoplasia encompasses a wide range of benign and malignant tumors, including sarcoids, melanomas, lymphomas, and more. Surgical management is often a vital aspect of treatment, either as a primary intervention or in conjunction with other modalities, such as chemotherapy or radiation therapy. This review aims to provide insights into the surgical management of equine neoplasia, considering the various tumor types, surgical planning, and techniques to improve cosmesis and outcomes.

PRINCIPLES OF SURGICAL ONCOLOGY

Surgical intervention is a key part of cancer treatment curing more solid tumors than any other modality. Indeed, approximately 60% of human patients that are cured of cancer are cured by surgery alone. The best chance to remove a tumor, to prevent recurrence, and to reduce complications, is the first surgical attempt. Historically, oncology surgery worked on the premise that increasingly radical surgery would result in higher cure rates.[1] However, in recent years a paradigm shift has been seen, with the recognition of the role of multimodal therapy, including (electro)chemotherapy or radiation therapy to reduce the requirement for, and detrimental effects of, radical surgery. The role of a surgeon in cancer treatment is constantly evolving with advances in surgical skills and experience playing a pivotal role.[2]

Equine Referral Hospital, Royal Veterinary College, Hawkshead Lane, North Mymms, Hatfield, Hertfordshire AL9 7TA, UK
E-mail address: afiskejackson@rvc.ac.uk

Vet Clin Equine 40 (2024) 371–385
https://doi.org/10.1016/j.cveq.2024.07.003   vetequine.theclinics.com
0749-0739/24/Crown Copyright © 2024 Published by Elsevier Inc. All rights reserved, including those for text and data mining, AI training, and similar technologies.

To transform into a cancerous cell, a normal cell undergoes a complex process of genetic alterations. This results in either loss of tumor inhibitory factors by tumor suppressor genes, such as p53, or activation of tumor-promoting factors via oncogenes (a mutated gene that has the potential to cause cancer). Activation of oncogenes can be caused by point mutations, gene amplification, or chromosome rearrangements.

These genotype alterations result in the phenotypic characteristics of tumors, which include the following:

1. Insensitivity to antigrowth signals
2. Unlimited replication
3. Evasion of apoptosis
4. Self-sufficient growth signals
5. Sustained angiogenesis
6. Tissue invasion and metastasis

The initiation of a cell's progression to a malignant phenotype occurs either via a genetic heritable mutation or, as in the case of chemical carcinogenesis, following exposure of a cell's DNA to a mutagen, resulting in base alterations in nuclear material. Next, the initiated cell must be exposed to a promoting agent if tumor growth is to occur. This will lead to lesions, such as papillomas or polyps. When a tumor develops the ability to undergo angiogenesis, local tissue invasion and metastasis to regional and distant sites progression will occur.

NEOADJUVANT THERAPY

Large tumors, or those adjacent to vital structures, can appear inoperable, at least to achieve a sufficient margin. Although neoadjuvant therapies are uncommon in veterinary medicine, consideration should be made as to whether a reduction in size could be achieved with chemotherapy. This has been shown to be beneficial in dogs with intermediate-grade mast cell tumors, where treatment with prednisolone resulted in tumor size reduction, allowing surgical excision with margins to be achieved.[3] Local chemotherapy can also be implemented following cytoreduction after a marginal excision of a malignant tumor.[4,5] Wound healing can be impaired with neoadjuvant therapies, and this should be considered and communicated to the owners.[6,7] Ideally, local chemotherapy would be administered once wound healing has been completed; this could be at the time of suture removal.

SURGICAL DOSE

When planning surgical excision of a tumor, the first consideration will be the surgical dose; this refers to how aggressive the excision needs to be with respect to the edges of the tumor. The surgical dose can be intracapsular (debulking), marginal, wide, or radical excisions.[8] An intracapsular excision involves disruption of the capsule, or pseudocapsule, of the organ in which the tumor is growing, allowing the tumor to be removed in pieces. A marginal excision is performed immediately outside the capsule or pseudocapsule so the tumor is "shelled out"; an example of this would be a benign dermal melanoma in the parotid region where wide surgical margins are impossible due to the proximity of vital structures.[5] A wide excision involves removal of the tumor alongside 2 to 3 cm of normal tissue surrounding it, or one fascial plane deep to cutaneous or subcutaneous tumors; the tumor capsule is not entered. The tumor margins created during surgical excision are based on imaging and/or palpation and do not necessarily represent the histologic margin. An example would be a mast cell tumor on the limb.[9] A radical excision involves removal of the entire structure in which the tumor is growing. Such excisions are less common in horses, unlike in small animals where limb amputations are ethically viable, but an example in the horse would be ovariohysterectomy to treat uterine neoplasia.[10] The most common error in surgical oncology is using too low a surgical dose for fear of not being able to close the resultant defect. However, it should be considered that it is better to leave a wound open than to leave tumor cells remaining.[11]

The goal of surgical excision will either be curative, palliative, or cytoreductive, and this will determine the surgical dose. Which of these goals is to be pursued will be determined by several factors. The first of these will be the type of tumor being treated. Benign tumors are contained in their capsule, therefore only requiring a marginal excision. Malignant tumors can extend into the surrounding tissue at the microscopic level, requiring a wide excision to be curative. However, if the goal with a malignant tumor is palliative or cytoreductive, a marginal excision can be performed. This can be combined with local adjunctive chemotherapy or radiotherapy. The decision to proceed with palliative or cytoreductive surgery should be discussed fully with the owner and should only be considered if the tumor is causing obstruction or functional problems for the horse. Where only a few tumor cells are left behind, local chemotherapy may be able to kill these remaining cells. Otherwise, palliation is likely to be only temporary and should only performed when absolutely necessary, as excessive bleeding and wound dehiscence can occur in such cases.

Other factors that determine the goal of the surgery are the tumor size and location, the stage of the cancer, overall health status of the patient, the risk of complications with the proposed excision, the prognosis, and the goals and expectations of the owners.

BIOPSY

Knowledge of the tumor type is essential to inform the surgeon on the most appropriate surgical dose and what the goal of the excision should be. There are several biopsy techniques available; the type chosen will depend on the tumor location, finances available, experience of the surgeon, and the suspected tumor type.

Fine needle aspiration is a minimally invasive technique that requires minimal equipment, can be performed with minimal patient discomfort, and can provide useful information before surgical excision. Imaging, such as ultrasonography, can be useful to guide the needle into the target tissue to ensure a representative sample is obtained. Often its goal is to differentiate between inflammatory and neoplasia tissue. If neoplastic tissue is present, the goal is to ascertain whether the tumor is benign or malignant. The results of a fine needle aspirate may confirm the presence of neoplastic tissue but not conclusively determine the tumor type. This would indicate the need for histopathology of a sample of tumor tissue. When comparing fine needle aspiration with histopathology, for cutaneous and subcutaneous masses, the agreement is generally good with a sensitivity of 89% and specificity of 98% for diagnosing neoplasia, although the numbers vary according to the tumor type.[12]

Needle core biopsies are useful to biopsy soft tissue masses with minimal additional equipment and low patient morbidity. Ultrasound guidance is recommended to ensure representative tissue is collected and to avoid vital structures such as large blood vessels.

A punch biopsy is a simple and effective method to sample cutaneous lesions. If the mass is subcutaneous, the overlying skin can be incised, and tissues can be dissected over the mass to allow collection of a more representative sample.

A wedge biopsy provides a larger sample of tissue than a punch or needle core biopsy, thereby maintaining more normal architecture of the biopsy tissue for histopathologic examination. The location of the biopsy should be such that any subsequent excision can easily include the biopsy site. Hematoma or seroma formation should be prevented, as it can risk seeding of tumor cells to the adjacent tissue. Although, historically, the best site was considered to be the junction between normal and abnormal tissue, modern practice recommends avoiding entering uninvolved tissue. A common error is to biopsy just the fibrous capsule surrounding the mass so the surgeon should ensure a sample of sufficient depth has been obtained. The risk of complications are higher than with needle core or punch biopsies and includes infection, hemorrhage, and swelling.

Excisional biopsies have the advantage of being both diagnostic and a treatment modality. However, the risk of an inappropriate treatment exists in the absence of a clear preoperative diagnosis with the high potential for doing too little, or too much, surgery. Excisional biopsies have been described as unplanned marginal resections, as they are performed without prior knowledge of the tumor type. The best time for complete excision is the time of the first surgical excision because following an excision the local anatomy is forever altered. The altered tissue planes can allow remaining tumor cells to invade deeper and wider, and subsequent scar tissue will also compromise future surgical attempts at excision. The tumor location is the single biggest determinant on whether an excisional biopsy is viable, with a small tumor on the trunk being more attractive to remove with an excisional biopsy than the same size mass on the distal limb.

STAGING

The results of the tumor biopsy will report its malignancy and the likelihood of tumor spread. Further diagnostic tests will then be indicated and may include hematology and biochemistry analysis, urinalysis, thoracic radiography and ultrasonography, abdominal ultrasonography, and a thorough palpation of local lymph nodes. This may uncover concomitant disease, which could influence the surgical plan and report the overall prognosis for the patient.[8]

TUMOR MARGINS

Historically, dogma has suggested that a generous margin is likely to be curative, but this is not always the case. Even extensive, complete margins do not always result in a cure. A recent study examining surgical tumor margins in human patients with oral squamous cell carcinomas found that, provided margins were simply greater than 1 mm, they can be appropriate and curative.[13] With the associated potential morbidity resulting from larger margins, close examination of historical doctrines regarding size or margins following tumor resection should be performed.

Surgical margins can also be affected by the choice of instrument used for resection. Monopolar cutting diathermy and coagulation diathermy both cause significant thermal damage to the resected tissue alongside denaturing of the underlying muscle.[14] The effect of laser excision has not been investigated, but it likely causes more thermal damage than a harmonic scalpel, which operates at 80°C.[13] The thermal necrosis associated with laser surgery can delay wound healing, reduce resistance to infection, and damage tissue samples, making assessment of surgical margins difficult or impossible.[15] When compared with diathermy, less tissue damage and contraction were seen when a harmonic scalpel or conventional scalpel was used to simulate tumor resection on pigs' tongues.[14] The harmonic scalpel uses high-frequency ultrasonic energy of approximately 55,000 Hz, which is converted to mechanical energy at an active blade. This blade vibrates against an inactive blade over an excursion of 50 to 100 μm. The hydrogen bonds in water are disrupted by the vibration but, critically, at a lower temperature than conventional diathermy; the result is a bloodless field, which improves accuracy and reduces surgery time.

One of the most common neoplasms in horses are cutaneous melanomas, most of which are benign. Usually these can be excised with very small margins using sharp dissection and primary closure (**Fig. 1**A–C). Alternatively, a diode laser can be used to excise all affected tissue with the site left to heal by second intention (**Fig. 2**A–D). Both of these surgical techniques can be performed under epidural anesthesia; postoperatively, a fecal-softening diet is required alongside appropriate pain relief to facilitate defecation.

Shrinkage of the tissue will occur following resection owing to intrinsic tissue characteristics; this can exceed 20%.[16,17] Additional shrinkage occurs during fixation in formalin, but this is less than the shrinkage seen following tumor excision.[17] These factors should be taken into consideration when interpreting tumor margins histopathologically. In addition, the quality of the margin may be more relevant than the quantity.[8]

Given tissue barriers, such as muscle, fascia, joint capsule, cartilage, and bone, are resistant to tumor infiltration, including a tissue barrier beyond the site of tumor attachment will be more effective than a larger tissue margin. However, although fascia is easily identifiable during surgery, it is difficult to discern as a distinct structure on histology. Therefore, margin interpretation involving fascia can be challenging during histopathologic examination. In addition, most solid tumors initially expand within their tissue of origin and grow along the lines of least resistance. This has led to the proposal of compartmental tumor excision for musculoskeletal sarcomas, whereby, for example, an entire muscle or muscle group is removed rather than circumferentially resecting en bloc.[18] This technique for tumor excision has been shown to reduce recurrence in some tumor types and should be considered in veterinary surgical oncology.[8]

SURGICAL PLANNING

Appropriate presurgical planning should be performed, particularly where multiple tumors are to be excised and, where an appropriate, a skin reconstruction technique

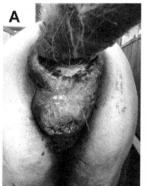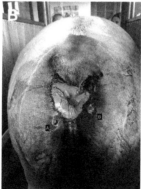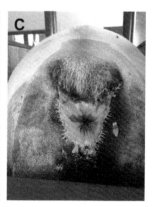

Fig. 1. (*A*) Huge dermal melanoma affecting the anus, perianal tissue, and tail dock. (*B*) Postoperative photograph showing an amputated tail and successful excision of the anal and perianal melanoma. Primary closure of the rectal mucosa to the skin has been performed apart from the region on the underside of the tail, which is too high-motion an area to allow primary closure. Sites "A" and "B" are previous drain holes. (*C*) Continued healing of the site with healthy granulation tissue present. (Courtesy images of Dr Liesbeth Haegeman, Equitom, Belgium.)

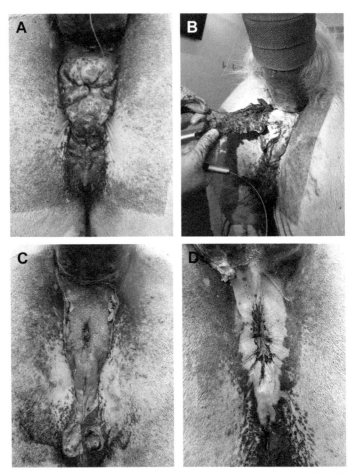

Fig. 2. (*A*) Dermal melanoma involving the anus, perianal tissue, and underside of the tail dock. (*B*) Intraoperative photograph showing the thin layer of cutaneous tissue being removed using a diode laser for successful marginal excision of the dermal melanomas. (*C*) Postoperative photograph showing a healthy bed of granulation tissue present during secondary intention healing of the site. (*D*) Completed healing of the site with unpigmented epithelium.

will need to be used. In addition, the order in which multiple tumors are to be excised should be considered; this should be in the order of benign tumors first progressing to malignant tumors. After each excision, new gloves, drapes, and instruments should be used to minimize the risk of tumor cells seeding into subsequent resections.

SURGICAL TECHNIQUES

Surgical excision of neoplasia is the treatment of choice especially if complete excision is possible and no metastasis has occurred. Consideration should be given of local vital structures, including blood vessels, nerves, lymph nodes, endocrine glands, and so forth, as well as locally relevant structures, such as the eye, oral cavity, rectum, and so forth. The proximity of these structures will dictate size of the margins that are possible; these will be considered against the recommended margins for the particular tumor type.[13,19] The aim is to achieve a result that is as functional and cosmetically acceptable as possible. The relative importance of the cosmetic outcome will vary depending on the use of the horse.

Incision orientation is important and should be dictated by the location, blood supply, and the extensibility of the skin. Elevating the skin over the tumor and assessing the tension during normal movement will report the extensibility of the skin. For tumors on the limb, incisions are usually best made parallel to the long axis of the limb to maintain blood supply and minimize tension. There are 2 types of tension acting on the skin: static skin tension, whereby the skin is clinging to the underlying body, and dynamic tension, which results from the pull of the underlying muscles. Static skin tension results from elastic fibers in the dermis and is the reason skin edges tend to retract when incised. Static (or relaxed) skin tension lines have been mapped,[20] but, ultimately, skin tension lines are heavily influenced by muscular contractions, movement over joints, and external forces. Nevertheless, making skin incisions parallel to these maximal lines of tension will result in reduced gapping, in reducing the propensity for tension on the wound edges (thereby reducing the likelihood of wound dehiscence), and will more likely heal with a smaller scar.

A fusiform skin incision will be commonly used to excise a tumor. To allow optimal closure of a fusiform incision, the length-to-width ratio should be 4:1 (**Fig. 3**A, B). Skin closure techniques (see later discussion) will be used to close the defect without tension.

Strict attention to hemostasis is important to prevent release of tumor cells into the circulation and to prevent hematoma formation. The lymph nodes that drain the tissue containing the tumor should be assessed and, ideally, biopsied. Lymph node biopsy is best achieved via an excisional biopsy, but incisional biopsies, fine needle aspirates, or needle core biopsies are often more prudent depending on the location of the lymph node.

Excision of a neoplastic mass will inevitably result in dead space and, potentially, skin loss; both must be managed appropriately to optimize resulting function and cosmesis. Failure to close dead space can result in formation of a hematoma or seroma; not only are these a good medium for bacterial growth but also they will place tension on the wound closure. Dead space can be managed in 4 ways depending on the location:

1. Placement of deep, buried sutures to appose anatomic layers. This can be using 2 barbed suture wound closure devices[21] or with other suture material. Buried sutures should be monofilament and absorbable and the smallest diameter possible,

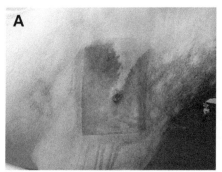
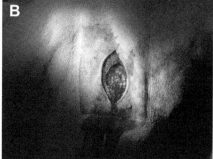

Fig. 3. (A) Benign, solitary, cutaneous nodular mast cell tumor on the shoulder of a horse. (B) A fusiform skin incision of a 4:1 length-to-width ratio, alongside one fascial plane deep margin, used to excise the tumor.

as excess suture used can potentiate infection.[22] Strict attention to Halsted's principles of gentle tissue handling, strict aseptic technique, sharp anatomic dissection of tissues, careful hemostasis, obliteration of dead space, and avoidance of tension, is also imperative.[23]

2. Passive or active drains remove fluid from the dead space, thereby reducing the pressure on the sutures and reducing the risk of infection (**Fig. 4**A, B). However, they can serve as a two-way street, allowing bacteria to enter the wound. Therefore, once drainage volume stops, or plateaus, the drain should be removed. Where there is a risk that the resection is incomplete, drains should be avoided, as they inevitably disrupt deep or lateral tissue planes seeding tumor cells along the drain path.

3. Mesh expansion of the skin (**Fig. 5**A–D) alongside, allowing mobilization of the skin to allow primary closure, also allows drainage of any accumulating fluid.

4. Where possible, appropriately applied pressure bandages can be used in combination with the above techniques, or alone, to reduce dead space. Care must be taken to avoid excessive pressure to ensure maintenance of blood supply to the wound.

SURGICAL TECHNICAL PRINCIPLES

There are specific measures the surgeon should take to reduce the risk of local or distant seeding of tumor cell and thereby increase the chances of a successful outcome:

1. The tumor should be handled as if it is an abscess to prevent exfoliation.

2. It should be draped off from the rest of the surgical field and isolated with moistened laparotomy sponges and, if required, manipulated with stay sutures or with atraumatic instruments placed in adjacent normal tissue.

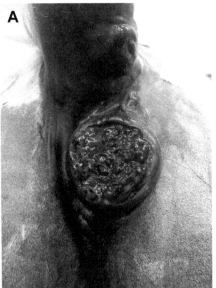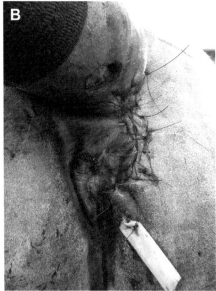

Fig. 4. (*A*) Large perianal ulcerated dermal melanoma with additional dermal melanoma on the ventral aspect of the dock. (*B*) Placement of a Penrose drain following excision of the melanoma to facilitate drainage from the resultant dead space. This was removed after 2 days. The melanoma on the ventral aspect of the dock has been removed using a diode laser.

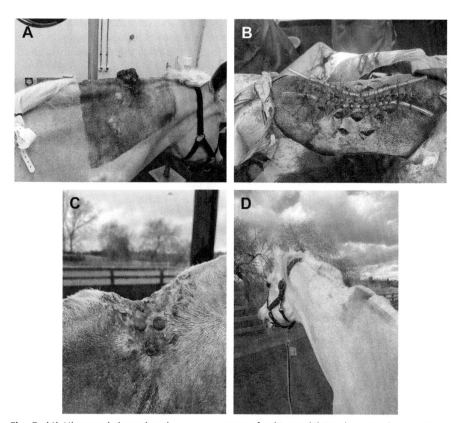

Fig. 5. (*A*) Ulcerated dermal melanoma on crest of a horse. (*B*) Mesh expanding incisions used alongside stented (tension-relieving) vertical mattress sutures to achieve closure of the defect following tumor excision. (*C*) Partial wound dehiscence occurred resulting in second-intention healing following formation of a healthy granulation bed. (*D*) Subsequent healing of the site with no tumor recurrence.

3. Sharp dissection is favored over blunt dissection, as it decreases the chances of leaving tumor cells and the likelihood of deviating from the preestablished margin.
4. Tumors can adhere to the surrounding structures without obvious evidence of invasion. However, in human oncology, such adhesions can represent tumor invasion in 57% of cases.[15] Therefore, structures adhered to tumors should be included in the excision, or at least an appropriate margin taken.
5. Monofilament suture material should be used for vessel ligation and wound closure, as multifilament sutures can trap tumor cells in the interstices of the braided material, risking local tumor recurrence.
6. Most local chemotherapy drugs are reported not to influence wound healing. However, if postoperative local chemotherapy is planned, it is prudent to use a monofilament absorbable suture that maintains its tensile strength for as long as possible, for example, polydioxanone.
7. No contact should be made with ulcerated or open areas of tumor with gloves or instruments.
8. Wound lavage following tumor excision is controversial, as it may disseminate any exfoliated cells throughout the lavaged cavity. In addition, tumor cells have been

shown to adhere to certain cellular receptors, and, in such cases, lavage has been shown to be ineffective. However, the known benefits of reducing tissue dehydration and removal of blood clots and any foreign material, thereby reducing infection, should also be considered.

9. Minimize tension on skin closures; patient positioning during surgery should be so the maximum tension on the skin is being exerted.

10. Use tension-relieving techniques, such as tension-relieving sutures and flaps during closure.[24,25]

11. Control of seroma or hematoma formation in dead space should be encouraged, as, if tumor excision is incomplete, tumor cells will spread widely, via the fluid, throughout the subcutaneous space during movement.

12. If a drain was placed following biopsy, the drain hole and biopsy tract must be removed en bloc with the tumor.

13. The pseudocapsule surrounding a tumor should not be penetrated; this is constructed of compressed tumor cells, which will seed easily to surround tissue.[24]

14. A new set of instruments, gloves, gowns, and drapes should be used to close the defect following tumor excision even during subsequent tumor removal on the same patient.

SKIN CLOSURE TECHNIQUES

Following excision of a tumor that involves the skin, the surgeon will be presented with the challenge of closing the skin while avoiding too much tension. Tension on suture lines results in ischemia of the wound edges, increased risk of scarring, and likely partial or complete wound dehiscence. Techniques to reduce tension include the use of tension-relieving suture patterns, undermining the surrounding skin, using tension-relieving incisions, or using skin mobilization techniques.

UNDERMINING THE SKIN

The simplest tension-relieving technique is undermining the skin edges around the excision site. The is best achieved using blunt dissection while being cognizant of the local neurovascular supply. Inserting Metzenbaum scissors closed into an appropriate fascial plane, followed by opening the blades, is the most commonly used method. Sharp dissection should only be used when necessary, in cases of chronic, fibrotic wounds, and even in such cases, a combination of sharp and blunt dissection techniques can be used. The depth of the dissection is determined by site, being below the panniculus muscle on the trunk and between the subcutaneous tissue and deep fascia on the limbs (where there is no panniculus muscle).[26] Drawing the skin together using towel clamps can guide the surgeon as to how far the skin needs to be undermined and whether persistent tension exists. Usually a distance equal to the width of the defect itself should be undermined on each side.[27] In chronic wounds, development of fibrous tissue leads to a loss of skin elasticity, potentially requiring more extensive undermining or other tension-relieving techniques.

TENSION-RELIEVING INCISIONS

Longitudinal incisions made adjacent to the wound edge with subsequent undermining of the tissue between the wound and the incision allows more movement of the skin than undermining alone. Such an incision can be made on one or both sides of the incision and can be targeted where needed. They should be made approximately the width of the wound away from the wound edge and are usually not closed. This technique can be used where it is necessary to provide skin coverage to a more vital area, such as a bone, tendon, or ligament.[27]

MESH EXPANSION

Mesh expansion is combined with undermining to mobilize skin for closure. Small incisions are made in undermined skin in staggered rows parallel to the wound edges; the rows of stab incisions should be approximately 1 cm apart (see **Fig. 5A–D**). This technique shows the more immediate effect in fresh incisions, but in chronic wounds, expansion of the skin can occur during subsequent hours through stress relaxation. An added benefit of this technique is the drainage afforded by the stab incisions.

Z-PLASTY

When faced with a large defect to close following tumor excision and where primary closure is essential, strategically placed incisions can allow relief of tension and closure; one such technique is a Z-plasty. Loose tissue is recruited from the sides of the surgical site, allowing transposition of the mobilized skin to where it is needed. A Z-shaped incision is made, and the 2 resultant triangular portions of skin are undermined. The incisions should be of the same length with, typically, an angle of 60° between them. The 2 triangular portions of skin are transposed; this can result in a 75% gain in length. A sliding Z-plasty is particularly useful when faced with reconstruction of the lateral canthus of the eye following tumor excision (**Fig. 6A–D**).[28,29] The tumor is fully excised using a square, or rhomboid, incision, and the surrounding skin and tarsoconjunctiva are undermined using bunt dissection. A triangle of skin is excised dorsal and ventral to the defect, allowing the skin to be advanced to cover the defect. The base of each triangle aligns with the diagonal of the defect. The eyelid margin at the lateral canthus is re-created by suturing the skin and conjunctiva together using 4-0 to 6-0 Polyglactin 910.[30]

PEDICLE FLAPS

A pedicle graft maintains its blood supply by virtue of its attachment on one of the short sides of the rectangle. A length-to-width ratio of 1.5:1 has been used successfully on the limb, while a length-to-width ration of 3:1 has been used successfully on the head. Flaps with a narrower base have greater maneuverability but a greater risk of compromised blood supply, whereas the reverse is true for a wide-based flap.[31,32]

Bipedicle flaps have the advantage of having 2 blood supplies, thereby ensuring survival of the mobilized skin. A skin incision is made parallel to the wound edge the same distance away as the width of the defect. The skin is undermined under the flap and surrounding skin so the original defect can be closed. The author prefers bipedicle flaps to single-pedicle flaps because of the superior blood supply and resultant improved survival of the flap.

SLIDING H-PLASTY

When faced with a rectangular defect following tumor excision, a sliding H-plasty can be used to advance adjacent skin to cover the defect. Two single-pedicle flaps can be made on each side so they joint in the middle, or one side can be advanced, for

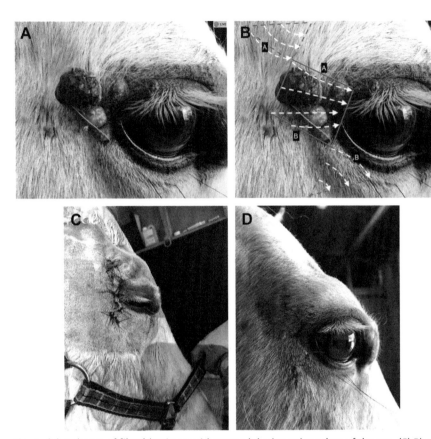

Fig. 6. (*A*) A cluster of fibroblastic sarcoids around the lateral canthus of the eye. (*B*) Planned incisions (*lines*) showing the central rectangle of skin containing the sarcoids to be excised, alongside the 2 triangles dorsally and ventrally. The surrounding skin is undermined, allowing mobilization of the skin in the direction of the arrows. Skin edges "A" are apposed, and skin edges "B" are apposed. (*C*) Immediately postoperative photograph showing successful excision of the cluster of sarcoids and reconstruction of the lateral canthus of the eye. (*D*) Successful healing of the surgical site with minimal scarring and no sarcoid recurrence. (Courtesy images of Safia Barakzai FRCVS, Equine Surgical Referrals, UK.)

example, a sliding H-plasty when removing an eyelid mass (**Fig. 7**A–E). Such a reconstructive procedure is required when greater than one-third of the eyelid margin has been lost. Slightly diverging vertical skin incisions are made as a continuation of the original excision, extending in length approximately twice the width of the eyelid margin defect; divergence will help to compensate for the consequent wound contracture. Advancement of the flap will cause laxity of skin on each side; triangular portions of skin ("Burow triangles") can be removed, thereby preventing formation of a dog-ear and reducing tension. Once the skin is advanced, the triangular defect is closed.[33] Given the anticipated wound contracture, advancing and suturing the flap a small distance beyond the eyelid margin will counter this. The flap is sutured to the conjunctiva at the eyelid margin, and to the adjacent skin, using 4-0 to 6-0 Polyglactin 910.[30]

There are numerous other reconstructive procedures, especially applicable to removal of tumors around the eye; these can be found in several other sources.[30,34,35]

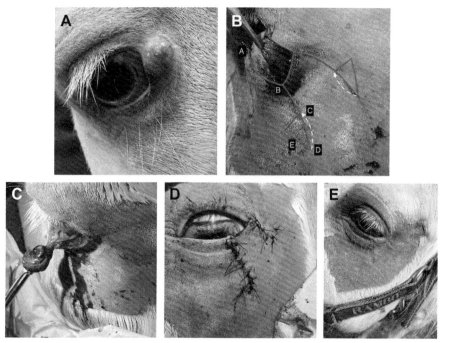

Fig. 7. (*A*) Nodular dermal melanoma on the ventrolateral aspect of the lower eyelid. (*B*) Planned incisions (*lines*; AB = BC = CD = DE), including the rectangular area to remove the melanoma and the 2 Burow triangles where the skin will be removed. The surrounding skin is undermined, allowing mobilization of the skin in the direction of the arrows. (*C*) First rectangular incision to remove the nodular dermal melanoma. (*D*) Immediate postoperative photograph showing successful reconstruction of the ventrolateral aspect of the lower eyelid. (*E*) Successful healing of the surgical site. (Courtesy images of Safia Barakzai FRCVS, Equine Surgical Referrals, UK.)

SUMMARY

Surgical management remains a critical component of the treatment of equine neoplasia, offering potential curative options for some tumor types. However, optimal outcomes require careful consideration of tumor characteristics and selection of the most appropriate surgical technique. As ongoing research continues to refine the understanding of equine neoplasia, veterinary surgeons can provide more effective and tailored treatment strategies for affected horses, ultimately improving their overall quality of life.

CLINICS CARE POINTS

- Preoperative biopsy guides the appropriate surgical dose required; benign tumors may only require a marginal excision.

- Neoadjunctive therapy following surgical excision has the potential to kill any remaining tumor cells.

- Numerous skin reconstruction techniques exist to allow closure of defects where healing by second intention is not viable, for example, around eyes.

- Fascial planes provide a robust barrier to tumor infiltration and should be borne in mind when planning a surgical excision of neoplasia.

DISCLOSURE

The author has nothing to disclose.

REFERENCES

1. Wyld L, Audisio RA, Poston GJ. The evolution of cancer surgery and future perspectives. Nat Rev Clin Oncol 2015;12(2):115–24.
2. Drixler TA, Voest EE, van Vroonhoven TJMV, et al. Angiogenesis and surgery: from mice to man. Eur J Surg 2000;166(6):435–46.
3. Stanclift RM, Gilson SD. Evaluation of neoadjuvant prednisone administration and surgical excision in treatment of cutaneous mast cell tumors in dogs. J Am Vet Med Assoc 2008;232(1):53–62.
4. Lowe R, Gavazza A, Impellizeri JA, et al. The treatment of canine mast cell tumours with electrochemotherapy with or without surgical excision. Vet Comp Oncol 2017;15(3):775–84.
5. Groom LM, Sullins KE. Surgical excision of large melanocytic tumours in grey horses: 38 cases (2001–2013). Equine Vet Educ 2018;30(8):438–43.
6. Cornell K, Waters DJ. Impaired wound healing in the cancer patient: effects of cytotoxic therapy and pharmacologic modulation by growth factors. Vet Clin North Am Small Anim Pract 1995;25(1):111–31.
7. Shamberger RC, Devereux DF, Brennan MF. The effect of chemotherapeutic agents on wound healing. Int Adv Surg Oncol 1981;4:15–58.
8. Culp WTN, Ehrhart N. Principles of surgical oncology. Vet Surg Oncol 2022;1–16.
9. Johnston GCA, Zedler ST. Treatment of an invasive equine mast cell tumour in the extensor carpi radialis by extensive tenomyectomy and local corticosteroid injections. Equine Vet Educ 2019;31(6):e34–8.
10. Santschi EM, Adams SB, Robertson JT, et al. Ovariohysterectomy in six mares. Vet Surg 1995;24(2):165–71.
11. Withrow SJ. Surgical oncology. Vet Q 1998;20(sup1):S12–3.
12. Ghisleni G, Roccabianca P, Ceruti R, et al. Correlation between fine-needle aspiration cytology and histopathology in the evaluation of cutaneous and subcutaneous masses from dogs and cats. Vet Clin Pathol 2006;35(1):24–30.
13. Brennan PA, Dylgjeri F, Coletta RD, et al. Surgical tumour margins and their significance in oral squamous cell carcinoma. J Oral Pathol Med 2022;51(4):311–4.
14. George KS, Hyde NC, Wilson P, et al. Does the method of resection affect the margins of tumours in the oral cavity? Prospective controlled study in pigs. Br J Oral Maxillofac Surg 2013;51(7):600–3.
15. Farese JP, Bacon NJ, Liptak JM, et al. Introduction to oncologic surgery for the general surgeon. In: Tobias KM, Johnston SA, editors. Veterinary surgery: small animal. St Louis (MO): Elsevier; 2012. p. 304–24.
16. Umstattd LA, Mills JC, Critchlow WA, et al. Shrinkage in oral squamous cell carcinoma: An analysis of tumor and margin measurements in vivo, post-resection, and post-formalin fixation. Am J Otolaryngol 2017;38(6):660–2.
17. Pangare TB, Waknis PP, Bawane SS, et al. Effect of formalin fixation on surgical margins in patients with oral squamous cell carcinoma. J Oral Maxillofac Surg 2017;75(6):1293–8.

18. Enneking WF. A system of staging musculoskeletal neoplasms. Clin Orthop Relat Res 1986;204:9–24.
19. Dickinson IC, Whitwell DJ, Battistuta D, et al. Surgical margin and its influence on survival in soft tissue sarcoma. ANZ J Surg 2006;76(3):104–9.
20. Wakuri H, Sakuma Y, Mutoh K, et al. Cleavage line patterns of the skin in the horse. Okajimas Folia Anat Jpn 1990;67(5):351–63.
21. Beggan CP, Quinn GC, D'Amours GH. Mammary tubulopapillary carcinoma in a mare, requiring bilateral mastectomy. N Z Vet J 2023;71(6):344–7.
22. de Holl D, Rodeheaver G, Edgerton MT, et al. Potentiation of infection by suture closure of dead space. Am J Surg 1974;127(6):716–20.
23. Thomas RJS. Principles of surgical oncology. In: Textbook of surgery. 3rd edition. Blackwell Publishing Ltd; 2008. p. 67–74.
24. Soderstrom MJ, Gilson SD. Principles of surgical oncology. Vet Clin North Am Small Anim Pract 1995;25(1):97–110.
25. Aiken SW. Principles of surgery for the cancer patient. Clin Tech Small Anim Pract 2003;18(2):75–81.
26. Swaim SF. Principles of plastic and reconstructive surgery. Textb small Anim Surg 1993;280–94.
27. Provost PJ, Bailey JV. Principles of plastic reconstructive surgery. In: Auer AA, Stick AA, editors. Equine surgery. 4th edition. St Louis (MO): Elsevier-Saunders; 2012. p. 271–84.
28. Stashak TS, Schumacher J. Principles and techniques for reconstructive surgery. Equine wound Manag 2016;200–30.
29. Jansson J, Knottenbelt D, Hennessy S. Use of random pattern skin flaps for wound closure in two horses. Equine Vet Educ 2022;34(2):e83–90.
30. Mowat FM, Bartoe JT. Adnexal surgery. In: Auer JA, Stick JA, Kummerle JM, et al, editors. Equine surgery. 5th edition. St Louis (MO): Elsevier; 2019. p. 927–56.
31. Hinchcliff KW, MACDONALD DR, Lindsay WA. Pedicle skin flaps in ponies: viable length is related to flap width. Equine Vet J 1992;24(1):26–9.
32. Madison JB, Donawick WJ, Johnston DE, et al. The use of skin expansion to repair cosmetic defects in animals. Vet Surg 1989;18(1):15–21.
33. Rose BL, Mair TS. Reconstructive blepharoplasty following eyelid melanoma excision using a sliding skin flap in six horses. Equine Vet Educ 2023;35(5):e406–13.
34. Giuliano EA. Equine ocular adnexal and nasolacrimal disease. In: Gilger BC, editor. Equine ophthalmology. 2nd edition. Elsevier Saunders; 2011. p. 133–80.
35. Gelatt KN. Diseases and surgery of the canine eyelid, . Gelatt KN vet ophthalmol. 4th edition. Ames: Iowa Blackwell Publ; 2007.

Chemotherapeutics in Equine Practice

Fernando Malalana, DVM, PhD, FHEA, FRCVS

KEYWORDS

- Horse • Tumor • Chemotherapy • Cytotoxic

KEY POINTS

- Chemotherapy is the treatment of cancerous cells through the use of cytotoxic drugs.
- Cytotoxic drugs preferentially target rapidly dividing cells, such as those in neoplastic tissues. However, they may also harm normal cells leading to adverse effects.
- The use of systemic (intravenous) chemotherapy in equine practice is generally limited to the management of lymphoma. This is probably due to the high costs of treatment and small number of suitable cases.
- Cytotoxic drugs are commonly used in the treatment of accessible skin tumors. These drugs can either be applied topically in the form of ointments or injected intralesionally.
- Cytotoxic drugs have been classified as carcinogenic, mutagenic, teratogenic, abortifacient, and increase the risk of stillbirth. Therefore, extreme caution should be followed when preparing, handling, administering, and disposing them.

DEFINITION, GENERAL PRINCIPLES, AND INDICATIONS

Chemotherapy is the treatment of cancerous cells through the use of cytotoxic drugs.[1] Chemotherapeutic agents typically damage DNA resulting in direct cell death, apoptosis, or inability to undergo mitosis.[2] These drugs preferentially target rapidly dividing cells, such as those in neoplastic tissues. However, chemotherapeutic drugs are non-specific and they may also harm normal cells, especially those in fast dividing tissues such as bone marrow, lymphoid cells, hair follicles, and enterocytes, leading to characteristic side effects (anemia, immunosuppression diarrhea, or hair loss).[1] In order to minimize the number and severity of adverse effects, in most chemotherapy regimens doses are administered at different intervals to provide drug-free periods for the normal tissues to recover.[1] It is important to note, however, that systemic chemotherapy protocols in domestic animals tend to be less aggressive than in people, with lower doses and longer treatment intervals, because prolonged survival with an acceptable quality of life, rather than complete cure, is the desired outcome in most

Philip Leverhulme Equine Hospital, University of Liverpool, Leahurst Campus, Chester High Road, Neston CH64 7TE, United Kingdom
E-mail address: f.malalana@liverpool.ac.uk

Vet Clin Equine 40 (2024) 387–395
https://doi.org/10.1016/j.cveq.2024.07.004
0749-0739/24/© 2024 Elsevier Inc. All rights reserved, including those for text and data mining, AI training, and similar technologies.
vetequine.theclinics.com

situations.[3] One way to minimize the adverse effects of chemotherapeutic drugs is the administration of metronomic chemotherapy, which has been described in horses. Metronomic chemotherapy is defined as the continuous administration of chemotherapy drugs but at doses lower than the conventional, maximally tolerated dose. This method of delivery inhibits tumor angiogenesis and modulates the immune system of the patient.[4]

Tumor growth is not constant. Initially, tumors grow exponentially over time and then rapidly plateau. Response to chemotherapy depends on which stage of growth the tumor is at, with those in the earlier, rapid growth phase showing greater response to these drugs. A major problem in the use of chemotherapy is that by the time a tumor is detected it has likely entered the plateau, slow growth phase.[5] Additionally, in larger tumors the deep cells may be protected by reduced blood and lymphatic supply, and increased intra-tumoral interstitial pressure, thus affecting the distribution of the drugs to the center of the tumor.[1]

The main indication for the use of chemotherapy is the treatment of tumors known to be sensitive to chemotherapeutic drugs (for example, lymphoma). However, in equine practice, chemotherapy is frequently administered in other situations such as to reduce the size of a tumor prior to surgical removal or to prevent recurrence after surgical excision or as palliative treatment to ease clinical signs until a defined goal (for example, foaling).[3,5]

MODES OF ACTION OF CHEMOTHERAPEUTIC AGENTS

Chemotherapeutic drugs can be classified according to their mechanism of action. However, some drugs have several mechanisms of action, and therefore, other classifications are possible, such as according to their metabolic targets (DNA, RNA, etc) or their spectrum (carcinoma, sarcoma, etc).[1,5]

Antimetabolites

Antimetabolites interfere with the synthesis of DNA by acting as structural analogues of purine and pyrimidine bases (or the corresponding nucleosides) or of folate cofactors, which are involved at several steps of purine and pyrimidine biosynthesis, preventing cell division.[6] Examples of antimetabolites are 5-Fluorouracil (5-FU), methotrexate, and cytosine arabinoside.

5-FU is metabolized into a nucleotide that is incorporated into RNA and ultimately interferes with DNA synthesis.[5] 5-FU is cell-cycle specific (S-phase); it inhibits DNA synthesis only in dividing cells so it may have lesser toxicity in quiescent cells.[7] There are reports on the use of 5-FU in horses for the treatment of sarcoids (topically and intralesionally) and squamous cell carcinomas (topically).[7–11]

Methotrexate inhibits dihydrofolic acid reductase, interfering with DNA synthesis, repair, and cellular replication.[5]

Cytosine arabinoside (cytarabine or ara-C) is a pyrimidine analog that is also cell-phase specific.[5] Systemic (intravenous) ara-C has been used in a number of combination protocols for the treatment of lymphoma in horses.[12]

Anti-tumour Antibiotics

Doxorubicin is an anti-tumour antibiotic derived from *Streptomyces* yeast species. It inhibits topoisomerase enzymes, responsible for the separation and re-attachment of DNA during replication, resulting in cell death during mitosis. In addition, it causes intercalation of DNA, leading to protein synthesis inhibition and free radical formation.[1,5] Intravenous doxorubicin has been used in horses for the treatment of lymphoma in combination with other drugs in a variety of protocols, but also as a sole agent for the treatment of sarcoids, melanomas, and carcinomas.[12,13]

Mitomycin C (MMC) is an antibiotic isolated from *Streptomyces caespitosus*. It is activated in the tissues to an alkylating agent that disrupts cancer cells by forming a complex with DNA. It also inhibits division of cancer cells by interfering with the biosynthesis of DNA. In addition, MMC reacts with oxygen to generate free radicals, causing cytotoxicity via lipid peroxydation, and DNA and protein damage.[14] Topical MMC has been commonly used for the management of ocular neoplasia in horses, mainly squamous cell carcinoma but also other ocular surface tumors such as melanoma, lymphoma, and hemangiosarcoma.[15–20] The use of MMC intralesionally for the treatment of sarcoids has also been described.[21,22]

Bleomycin is a water-soluble glycopeptide antibiotic isolated from *Streptomyces verticillus*. It interacts with DNA to cause both single and double strand damage. In the presence of oxygen, it generates local high concentrations of hydroxyl radicals that cause significant double-strand breaks.[23] There are reports on the use of topical and intralesional bleomycin for the treatment of sarcoids in horses.[23,24]

Actinomycin D (or Dactinomycin) is an antibiotic also isolated from *Streptomyces* species. It inhibits transcription by binding DNA at the transcription initiation complex and preventing elongation of RNA chain by RNA polymerase.[25]

Alkylating Agents

Alkylating agents bind DNA strands and change their structure, thus interfering with transcription, replication, and repair mechanisms. They inhibit DNA, RNA, and protein synthesis. These drugs are cell cycle phase non-specific.[5]

Cisplatin and Carboplatin are platinum-containing compounds that bind to DNA causing cross-linking, inhibiting protein synthesis, and ultimately leading to cell death.[5,26] Intralesional cisplatin and carboplatin have been used extensively for the treatment of sarcoids, but also other tumors, including sarcomas, melanomas, and hemangiosarcomas.[10,24,26–29]

Other examples of alkylating agents, which use has been described in horses are cyclophosphamide (intravenously), chlorambucil (orally), and Lomustine (CCNU) (intragastrically).[4,12]

Antitubulin Agents

Vincristine and Vinblastine are plant alkaloids that inhibit intracellular microtubule formation, an important part of the mitotic spindle formation, during metaphase. Vinblastine, in addition, interferes with amino acid metabolism.[5] Intravenous vincristine has been used in equine lymphoma cases.[12]

Miscellaneous Agents

L-asparaginase is a bacterium derived enzyme that degrades the amino acid asparagine inhibiting protein synthesis. Its use has been reported in the treatment of equine lymphoma (intramuscularly and subcutaneously).[12]

Others

Heavy metals (in particular arsenic) can induce apoptosis and have been shown to have anti-tumour effects in some cancer line cells. Both arsenic and zinc have been used topically for the treatment of sarcoids.[1]

Corticosteroids such as prednisolone and dexamethasone are commonly administered systemically during treatment of lymphoma in horses, but their intralesional uses have also been reported in mast cell tumors.[12,30] Corticosteroids bind to cytoplasmic receptors and inhibit DNA synthesis. However, their effect on equine lymphoma cases has not been definitively evaluated, and it may be that some of their perceived benefits are simply due to their effect to the inflammatory processes associated with some neoplasias.[1]

The expression of the enzyme Cyclooxygenase-2 (COX-2) has been documented in some equine tumors, mainly squamous cell carcinomas, but also in melanomas.[31–36] This has led to the use of *COX-2 inhibitors*, such as piroxicam and meloxicam, as adjunctive medication for a management of a small number of equine carcinoma cases.[4,37]

The histamine H2-receptor antagonist *cimetidine* has been found to be an effective chemotherapeutic agent in a number of human tumors due to inhibition of suppressor T cells and enhancement of Natural Killer cell activity.[1] The successful use of oral cimetidine for the treatment of melanoma was reported in a small case series of 3 horses. However, more recent studies have failed to replicate similar results.[38,39]

Imiquimod is an immune response modifier with antitumour effects through induction of cytokines and enhancement of cell-mediated cytolytic activity that has been used topically for the treatment of sarcoids.[40,41]

European mistletoe (*Viscum album austriacus*) aqueous extracts have been used as adjuvant in the treatment of a number of human cancers. Their antitumoural effects are mainly attributed to mistletoe lectins and viscotoxins, with cytotoxic and growth-inhibiting properties, in addition to immune modulating activity. A study assessed its efficacy for the management of sarcoids.[42] However, a recent randomized placebo-controlled double-blinded study assessing the efficacy of oral and subcutaneous mistletoe extract for the treatment of sarcoids failed to show any significant effect.[43]

ROUTES OF ADMINISTRATION
Systemic

The use of systemic (intravenous) chemotherapy in the treatment of cancer in horses has found only limited application. This is due to the small number of suitable cases, costs, and the logistics involved with the treatment processes. The major indication for the use of systemic chemotherapy in horses is in the treatment of lymphoma.[3,12]

A number of chemotherapeutic protocols for the treatment of lymphoma in horses have been described. Multiple-drug protocols are typically employed to minimize the possibility of acquired drug resistance by the tumoural cells.[3] Dosages are calculated on a square meter basis using the formula.[2]

Body surface area (m^2) = weight (g$^{2/3}$) x 10.5/10^4

The following drugs have been reported in horses (**Table 1**):[2,3,12]

Protocols described range from administration of a single drug to combinations of up to 5 different drugs. Perhaps the most common induction protocol reported for the treatment of lymphoma in horses involves administration of cyclophosphamide, cytosine arabinoside, and prednisolone. If remission is achieved, then the treatment intervals for each drug are increased.

In a recent study on the use of chemotherapy in 15 horses affected by lymphoma, complete remission was achieved in a third of the cases and partial remission in 60%, with an overall response rate of 93.3%. Median survival time was 8 months (range 1–46 months).[12] Adverse effects observed following the administration of this drugs are variable and include alopecia, neutropenia, lymphopenia, lethargy, neurotoxicity, and colic and hypersensitivity reactions. The worst side effects were associated with Doxorubicin. A case of sudden death occurred in one case 18 hours post-doxorubicin administration. Horses receiving systemic chemotherapy should be monitored for signs

Table 1
Square meter-based dosage calculation formula utilized to minimize the possibility of drug resistance

Drug	Dose	Frequency
Doxorubicin	35–70 mg/m^2 IV	Every 2–3 wk
Vincristine	0.55–0.7 mg/m^2 IV	Weekly
L-asparaginase	10,000–40,000 IU/m^2 IM or SC	Every 2–3 wk
Lomustine	65 mg/m^2 intragastrically	
Cyclosphosphamide	200 mg/m^2 IV	Every 1–2 wk
Cytosine arabinoside	175–300 mg/m^2 IV	Every 1–2 wk
Prednisolone	0.5–1 mg/Kg PO	Daily or every other d
Chlorambucil	20–30 mg/m^2 PO	Every 2 wk
Actinomycin-D	0.5–0.75 mg/m^2 IV	Every 3 wk

of gastrointestinal, renal, or neurologic toxicity. In addition, regular hematologic and serum biochemical evaluations, such as renal and hepatic markers, and red cell, white cell, and platelet counts, are advised.[12]

Local

Skin tumors make the greatest proportion of cancers seen in equine practice.[44–48] Local chemotherapy can be applied in cases where there is direct access to the tumor. This allows to improve the safety and reduce the costs and adverse effects associated with the treatment with chemotherapeutic agents.[1]

Topical

Chemotherapy agents in the form of ointments can be applied on accessible, superficial skin tumors. These treatments tend to be cheaper and easier to apply. However, there are important drawbacks that have to be taken into consideration when contemplating this form of treatment. Firstly, there is the risk of spread of the product applied to the healthy skin around the tumor. Similarly, due to their superficial application, there is also a risk of the product getting in contact with the human handlers. And finally, there is limited absorption of the product, generally restricting the application of this treatment modality to tumors less than 5 mm deep.[1] Products applied in this manner include 5-FU, Bleomycin, Imiquimod, and so forth.[1,8,23,41]

Intralesional

Injecting the chemotherapeutic agent directly into the tumor is a popular method of treatment for accessible skin neoplasia. This is a cost-effective method that allows higher concentrations of cytotoxic drugs to be achieved and increases the accuracy of the application whilst reducing the risk of accidental contact with the drug by the horse handler.[1] The type of formulation is important: aqueous solutions may diffuse from the tumor and be cleared within minutes, reducing its efficacy; therefore, the use of oil emulsions is recommended.[1] There are a number of examples of drugs used in this manner, including 5-FU, cisplatin, or Bleomycin.[11,24,27] Another alternative is the use of biodegradable beads impregnated in a chemotherapeutic agent that can be implanted within the tumor.[49,50]

Electrochemotherapy is a modality of treatment that combines the administration of intralesional chemotherapy with the direct application of short, intense electric pulses to the tumor. This increases the permeability of the cell membrane allowing the transport of molecules with poor membrane permeability, such as cisplatin, carboplatin, or bleomycin, into the tumor. In addition, it causes local vasoconstriction leading to drug sequestration.[26,51–53] This technique; however, has some disadvantages that may limit its application. The intense electric pulses cause profound discomfort and therefore this method of treatment requires general anesthesia. In addition, multiple treatments (4 on average) are required at 2-weekly intervals, increasing the costs and the risk of catastrophic injury associated with the repeated general anesthesia events.

HEALTH AND SAFETY ASPECTS

Cytotoxic drugs have been classified as carcinogenic, mutagenic, teratogenic, abortifacient, and increase the risk of stillbirth. Only trained personnel should handle, prepare, and administer chemotherapeutics to avoid any accidental exposure to these drugs. Likewise, precautions should be taken by owners handling horses undergoing chemotherapy or administering drugs to their horses.

Written policies and procedures for the safe handling of cytotoxic drugs must be in place in any facility in which chemotherapeutic agents are handled. Workers must be trained to wear appropriate personal protective equipment (PPE) and this should include chemotherapy-rated double gloving, long sleeve impermeable gown with back closure, shoe covers, and face shields.

Likewise, all employees should be aware of policies and procedures regarding spillages and the appropriate cleaning protocols.

The storage of these drugs should be carried out according to label recommendations. Cytotoxic drugs should be stored in a separate, dedicated area with clear signage. No food or drink should be consumed within this area.

Preparation of the drugs should be carried out in a vertical laminar flow cabinet with high-efficiency filtration. The preparation area should be clutter-free and contain only the necessary equipment, which should be gathered beforehand to avoid excess movement.

Two people should be present when administering chemotherapy to a horse. If the horse is uncooperative chemical restraint should be used. When administering intravenous chemotherapy, intravenous catheter must be placed. Once finished, the catheter should be removed and all material should be properly disposed according to local rules, by licensed cytotoxic waste disposal companies.

The excretion times of cytotoxic drugs have not been established in equine patients for most drugs, therefore the exact level of risk from exposure to excreted products is unknown. Typically, drugs can be found in the urine of treated animals for weeks after administration, although concentrations are markedly reduced after 3 days; likewise, many drugs can also be found in the feces for 5 to 7 days. Minimizing contact and the wearing of PPE by workers responsible for handling the horses and cleaning the stables is advisable. Likewise, clear written instructions including information about the safe handling of their horse should be provided to owners.[54]

CLINICS CARE POINTS

- The dose of the drug to be administered should be accurately calculated.
- The preparation and administration of cytotoxic agents should only be carried out by trained personnel, following approved policies and procedures on the safe handling these drugs.
- Two people should be present when administering chemotherapy to a horse, and sedative drugs should be used if the horse is uncooperative.

- All waste material, including catheters and administration lines, should be adequately disposed according to local rules.
- PPE should be worn for 5-7 days when handling horses that have received chemotherapy, as well as when cleaning their stable.

DISCLOSURE

The author declares no conflicts of interest.

REFERENCES

1. Knottenbelt DC, Patterson-Kane JC, Snalune KL. Principles of oncological therapy. In: Knottenbelt DC, Patterson-Kane JC, Snalune KL, editors. Clinical equine Oncology. 1st edition. Elsevier; 2015. p. 118-97.
2. Mair TS, Couto CG. The use of cytotoxic drugs in equine practice. Equine Vet Educ 2006;18(3):149-56.
3. Burns TA, Couto CG. Systemic chemotherapy for oncologic diseases. In: Robinson NE, Sprayberry KA, editors. Current therapy in equine medicine. 6th edition. St Louis: Saunders Elsevier; 2009. p. 15-8.
4. Tornago R, Sabattini S, De Simoi A, et al. Treatment of oral squamous cell carcinoma in a horse by surgical debulking followed by metronomic chemotherapy. Equine Vet Educ 2017;29:208-12.
5. Chun R, Garrett LD, Vail DM. Cancer chemotherapy. In: Withrow SJ, Vail DM, editors. Small animal clinical oncology. 4th edition. St Louis: Saunders Elsevier; 2007. p. 163-92.
6. Lansiaux A. Antimetabolites. Bull Cancer 2011;98(11):1263-74.
7. Offer KS, Marchesi F, Sutton DGM. Topical 5-fluorouracil as an adjunct treatment in equine corneolimbal squamous cell carcinoma. Equine Vet Educ 2022;34(9): e363-8.
8. Fortier LA, Macharg MA. Topical use of 5-fluorouracil for treatment of squamous-cell carcinoma of the external genitalia of horses - 11 cases (1988-1992). J Am Vet Med Assoc 1994;205:1183-5.
9. Paterson S. Treatment of superficial ulcerative squamous cell carcinoma in three horses with topical 5-fluorouracil. Vet Rec 1997;141:626-8.
10. Knottenbelt DC, Kelly DF. The diagnosis and treatment of periorbital sarcoid in the horse: 445 cases from 1974 to 1999. Vet Ophthalmol 2000;3:169-91.
11. Stewart AA, Rush B, Davis E. The efficacy of intratumoural 5-fluorouracil for the treatment of equine sarcoids. Aust Vet J 2006;84:101-6.
12. Luethy D, Frimberger AE, Bedenice D, et al. Retrospective evaluation of clinical outcome after chemotherapy for lymphoma in 15 equids (1991-2017). J Vet Intern Med 2019;33(2):953-60.
13. Théon AP, Pusterla N, Magdesian KG, et al. Phase I dose escalation of doxorubicin chemotherapy in tumor-bearing equidae. J Vet Intern Med 2013;27(5):1209-17.
14. Abraham IM, Selva D, CassonR Leibovitch I. Mitomycin - Clinical applications in ophthalmic practice. Drugs 2006;66:321-40.
15. Rayner SG, Van Zyl N. The use of mitomycin C as an adjunctive treatment for equine ocular squamous cell carcinoma. Aust Vet J 2006;84(1-2):43-6.
16. Malalana F, Knottenbelt DC, McKane SA. Mitomycin C, with or without surgery, for the treatment of ocular squamous cell carcinoma in horses. Vet Rec 2010; 167(10):373-6.

17. Clode AB, Miller C, McMullen RJ Jr, et al. A retrospective comparison of surgical removal and subsequent CO2 laser ablation versus topical administration of mitomycin C as therapy for equine corneolimbal squamous cell carcinoma. Vet Ophthalmol 2012;15(4):254–62.

18. Vallone LV, Neaderland MH, Ledbetter EC, et al. Suspected malignant transformation of B lymphocytes in the equine cornea from immune-mediated keratitis. Vet Ophthalmol 2016;19(2):172–9.

19. Scherrer NM, Lassaline M, Engiles J. Ocular and periocular hemangiosarcoma in six horses. Vet Ophthalmol 2018;21(4):432–7.

20. Strauss RA, Allbaugh RA, Haynes J, et al. Primary corneal malignant melanoma in a horse. Equine Vet Educ 2019;31:403–9.

21. Malalana F, Morgan RA, Knottenbelt DC, et al. Intralesional Mitomycin C for the treatment of periocular sarcoids. 2010. 49th BEVA Congress; Birmingham, UK, September 2010.

22. McKane SA and Coomer RP. A practical protocol for the clinical use of Mitomycin-C in the treatment of sarcoids in horses. 2013. 6th Congress of the European College of Equine Internal Medicine; Le Touquet, France, February 2013.

23. Knottenbelt DC, Watson AH, Hotchkiss JW, et al. A pilot study on the use of ultradeformable liposomes containing bleomycin in the treatment of equine sarcoid. Equine Vet Educ 2020;32:258–63.

24. Théon AP, Pascoe JR, Madigan JE, et al. Comparison of intratumoral administration of cisplatin versus bleomycin for treatment of periocular squamous cell carcinomas in horses. Am J Vet Res 1997;58(4):431–6.

25. Sobell HM. Actinomycin and DNA transcription. Proc Natl Acad Sci U S A 1985; 82(16):5328–31.

26. Tamzali Y, Borde I, Rols MP, et al. Successful treatment of equine sarcoids with cisplatin electrochemotherapy: A retrospective study of 48 cases. Equine Vet J 2012;44:214–20.

27. Théon AP, Wilson WD, Magdesian KG, et al. Long-term outcome associated with intratumoral chemotherapy with cisplatin for cutaneous tumors in equidae: 573 cases (1995-2004). J Am Vet Med Assoc 2007;230(10):1506–13.

28. Haspeslagh M, Vlaminck LE, Martens AM. Treatment of sarcoids in equids: 230 cases (2008-2013). J Am Vet Med Assoc 2016;249(3):311–8.

29. Norton AM, McGilp D, Vasey JR. Use of intralesional cisplatin to successfully treat distal limb haemangiosarcoma in a foal. Aust Vet J 2023;101(8):308–12.

30. Johnston GCA, Zedler ST. Treatment of an invasive equine mast cell tumour in the extensor carpi radialis by extensive tenomyectomy and local corticosteroid injections. Equine Vet Educ 2019;31:e34–8.

31. Elce YA, Orsini JA, Blikslager AT. Expression of cyclooxygenase-1 and -2 in naturally occurring squamous cell carcinomas in horses. Am J Vet Res 2007;68(1): 76–80.

32. McInnis CL, Giuliano EA, Johnson PJ, et al. Immunohistochemical evaluation of cyclooxygenase expression in corneal squamous cell carcinoma in horses. Am J Vet Res 2007;68(2):165–70.

33. Rassnick KM, Njaa BL. Cyclooxygenase-2 immunoreactivity in equine ocular squamous-cell carcinoma. J Vet Diagn Invest 2007;19(4):436–9.

34. Thamm DH, Ehrhart EJ 3rd, Charles JB, et al. Cyclooxygenase-2 expression in equine tumors. Vet Pathol 2008;45(6):825–8.

35. Smith KM, Scase TJ, Miller JL, et al. Expression of cyclooxygenase-2 by equine ocular and adnexal squamous cell carcinomas. Vet Ophthalmol 2008;11(Suppl 1):8–14.

36. van den Top JG, Harkema L, Ensink JM, et al. Expression of cyclo-oxygenases-1 and -2, and microsomal prostaglandin E synthase-1 in penile and preputial papillomas and squamous cell carcinomas in the horse. Equine Vet J 2014;46(5): 618–24.
37. Moore AS, Beam SL, Rassnick KM, et al. Long-term control of mucocutaneous squamous cell carcinoma and metastases in a horse using piroxicam. Equine Vet J 2003;35(7):715–8.
38. Goetz TE, Ogilvie GK, Keegan KG, et al. Cimetidine for treatment of melanomas in three horses. J Am Vet Med Assoc 1990;196(3):449–52.
39. Laus F, cerquetella M, Paggi E, et al. Evaluation of cimetidine as a therapy for dermal melanomatosis in grey horse. Isr J Vet Med 2010;65(2):48–52.
40. Sauder DN. Immunomodulatory and pharmacologic properties of imiquimod. J Am Acad Dermatol 2000;43(1 Pt 2):S6–11.
41. Nogueira SA, Torres SM, Malone ED, et al. Efficacy of imiquimod 5% cream in the treatment of equine sarcoids: a pilot study. Vet Dermatol 2006;17(4):259–65.
42. Christen-Clottu O, Klocke P, Burger D, et al. Treatment of clinically diagnosed equine sarcoid with a mistletoe extract (Viscum album austriacus). J Vet Intern Med 2010-Dec;24(6):1483–9.
43. Beermann A, Clottu O, Reif M, et al. A randomized placebo-controlled double-blinded study comparing oral and subcutaneous administration of mistletoe extract for the treatment of equine sarcoid disease. J Vet Intern Med 2024;26. https://doi.org/10.1111/jvim.17052. Epub ahead of print. PMID: 38529853.
44. Baker JR, Leyland A. Histological survey of tumours of the horse, with particular reference to those of the skin. Vet Rec 1975;96(19):419–22.
45. Sundberg JP, Burnstein T, Page EH, et al. Neoplasms of equidae. J Am Vet Med Assoc 1977;170(2):150–2.
46. Pascoe RR, Summers PM. Clinical survey of tumours and tumour-like lesions in horses in south east Queensland. Equine Vet J 1981;13(4):235–9.
47. Bastianello SS. A survey on neoplasia in domestic species over a 40-year period from 1935 to 1974 in the Republic of South Africa. IV. Tumours occurring in Equidae. Onderstepoort J Vet Res 1983;50(2):91–6.
48. Knowles EJ, Tremaine WH, Pearson GR, et al. A database survey of equine tumours in the United Kingdom. Equine Vet J 2016;48(3):280–4.
49. Hewes CA, Sullins KE. Use of cisplatin-containing biodegradable beads for treatment of cutaneous neoplasia in equidae: 59 cases (2000-2004). J Am Vet Med Assoc 2006;229:1617–22.
50. Marble GP, Sullins KE, Powers BK. Evaluation of a subcutaneously implanted biodegradable matrix with and without cisplatin in horses. Equine Vet Educ 2023; 35:e131–7.
51. Cemazar M, Tamzali Y, Sersa G, et al. Electrochemotherapy in veterinary oncology. J Vet Intern Med 2008;22(4):826–31.
52. Tozon N, Kramaric P, Kos Kadunc V, et al. Electrochemotherapy as a single or adjuvant treatment to surgery of cutaneous sarcoid tumours in horses: a 31-case retrospective study. Vet Rec 2016;179(24):627.
53. Souza C, Villarino NF, Farnsworth K, et al. Enhanced cytotoxicity of bleomycin, cisplatin, and carboplatin on equine sarcoid cells following electroporation-mediated delivery in vitro. J Vet Pharmacol Therapeut 2017;40(1):97–100.
54. Smith AN, Klahn S, Phillips B, et al. ACVIM small animal consensus statement on safe use of cytotoxic chemotherapeutics in veterinary practice. J Vet Intern Med 2018;32(3):904–13.

Radiotherapy in Equine Practice

Margaret C. Mudge, VMD*, Eric Green, DVM

KEYWORDS

- Horse • Radiation • Teletherapy • Sarcoid • Carcinoma

KEY POINTS

- Radiation therapy techniques for horses include teletherapy, brachytherapy, and plesiotherapy.
- Teletherapy with a linear accelerator is an effective treatment modality for many types of tumors of the equine head and distal limbs.
- Radiation therapy should be considered for tumors near joints, eyes, or other areas where large surgical margins would be difficult to achieve, and can be used as adjunctive therapy for many tumor types.
- Ideally the surgeon and radiation oncologist work together to determine a plan for tumor management and to advise the client on expectations and prognosis.

INTRODUCTION

Management of tumors in horses can be challenging, especially when there is a high risk of recurrence or when wide surgical excision would have unacceptable consequences based on damage to vital structures. Radiotherapy can be an effective treatment option or adjunct to surgical removal or debulking of the tumor. Radiotherapy has been described extensively in the small animal veterinary literature. A 2010 survey described radiation therapy facilities in the United States, Canada, and Europe; however, this survey did not address large animal patients or protocols.[1] Radiation therapy facilities that can accommodate large animals are limited, but there is evidence for efficacy of various types of radiotherapy in horses. The biologic action and types of radiation will be reviewed, with a focus on linear accelerator teletherapy. Management of the equine radiation patient and a review of the evidence for radiotherapy for specific tumor types in horses will then be discussed.

Department of Veterinary Clinical Sciences, The Ohio State University, The Ohio State University Veterinary Medical Center, 601 Vernon Tharp Street, Columbus, OH 43210, USA
* Corresponding author.
E-mail address: mudge.3@osu.edu

Vet Clin Equine 40 (2024) 397–408
https://doi.org/10.1016/j.cveq.2024.07.005
0749-0739/24/© 2024 Elsevier Inc. All rights reserved, including those for text and data mining, AI training, and similar technologies.
vetequine.theclinics.com

BIOLOGIC ACTION OF RADIATION

Radiation therapy, or radiotherapy, uses ionizing radiation in the form of high-energy photons or electrons to create DNA damage in cells. The radiation ionizes cells in the patient, liberating electrons from their orbits. The liberated electrons will interact directly with the DNA to create damage or with water molecules to create free radicals that cause the DNA damage. This damage is typically in the form of single-stranded and double-stranded DNA breaks that can lead to tumor and normal cell death during mitosis. Single-stranded DNA breaks can be repaired if the cells have sufficient time between mitotic events, often as little as 6 hours. As such, rapidly dividing normal and tumor cells experience more cell death due to lack of time available for repair before the next mitotic event. Radiation exposure essentially creates the same amount of DNA damage in a given cell regardless of the cell type. Fortunately, tumor cells are less effective at DNA repair than normal cells. This fact is exploited by radiotherapy protocols, which deliver smaller doses of radiation at regular intervals, often daily or every other day. This allows normal cells to repair most of their DNA damage between radiation doses while there is a gradual accumulation of unrepaired DNA damage in tumor cells. This results in a greater number of tumor cells dying than normal cells. The goal of radiotherapy is to deliver a total dose of radiation high enough to result in extensive tumor cell death, but not unacceptable normal cell death and the associated side effects.

TYPES OF RADIOTHERAPY

Radiotherapy can be delivered through several different methods: teletherapy, brachytherapy, and plesiotherapy.

Teletherapy (*tele* from the Greek *tēle* meaning "far off") uses a linear accelerator to deliver external beam radiation from a distance. Linear accelerators are large machines that generate high-energy photons or electrons that are directed at a patient positioned on a supporting couch. The machine emits radiation from a gantry and can rotate around a central point, called the isocenter, to treat the patient from any desired direction. Linear accelerators also have the capability of imaging the patient, either by creating a radiograph or computed tomographic (CT) images of the area treated to assure accurate patient positioning. Because of the high-energy radiation output, linear accelerators are housed within rooms with thick shielded walls (vaults or bunkers) and twisting entry hallways (mazes). For all veterinary patients, teletherapy requires general anesthesia as the patients must remain still during treatment and can only be monitored remotely from outside the vault.

Brachytherapy (*brachy* from the Greek *brachys* meaning "short") involves the implantation of radioactive seeds (typically iridium-192, iodine-125, palladium-103) smaller than a grain of rice into the tumor either individually or arranged within tubes where they constantly deliver a low dose rate of radiation. When placed individually, the seeds are left in permanently. When placed in tubes to deliver low dose rate brachytherapy, the tubes and seeds are removed when the desired total dose has been achieved, typically about 5 to 7 days. While the seeds are in place, the patients are radioactive and personnel and owner exposure to them must be limited until the seeds have decayed sufficiently to be safe or are removed. A way to avoid potential radiation exposure is to use a form of brachytherapy termed high dose rate brachytherapy. This involves the implantation of the tubes in the tumor and uses an external machine to push a high dose rate radiation source through the tubes, pausing at specific locations, delivering the desired dose of radiation in several sessions, rather than continuously over a week, similar to an external beam fractionated radiation therapy protocol. The duration of each session is dictated by the size of the area treated (number and length of the tubes) and the dose delivered. The tubes remain in place between sessions, but the patient is not radioactive as the radioactive source is housed in the external machine. Depending on the tumor location and the horse's temperament, brachytherapy can be performed under standing sedation and local anesthesia. Brachytherapy is limited to facilities specifically licensed to handle the radioactive material used.

Plesiotherapy (*plesio* from the Greek *plēsio* meaning "near") is a type of radiotherapy that is delivered by direct application of a mold or plaque customized specifically to the tumor shape. The plaque can be embedded with beta or gamma-ray sources (cesium-137, iridium-192, gold-198, iodine-125, ruthenium-106, cobalt-60, or palladium-103) to suit the desired depth of treatment. In veterinary medicine, to avoid the creation of custom plaques, a 1 cm diameter probe with embedded strontium-90 is often used. Strontium-90 has a half-life of 28.8 years and during radioactive decay, releases electrons that penetrate a few millimeters in tissue. This type of radiation is suitable for the treatment of small superficial tumors, ideally less than 1 cm in diameter and less than 3 mm thick, due to the size of the probe face and the depth of penetration of the radiation. Plesiotherapy is commonly used to treat small ocular tumors in small animal and equine patients and superficial cutaneous tumors in small animal patients. The duration of treatment is dependent on the radioactivity of the probe and may take several minutes so sedation is necessary in equine patients and general anesthesia is often used in small animal patients.

This article focuses on teletherapy treatment of equine tumors.

LINEAR ACCELERATOR-BASED TELETHERAPY TECHNIQUES

Delivery of radiation using a linear accelerator can be performed utilizing several different techniques. The choice of technique depends on the tumor size and location.

Electron Therapy

Superficial tumors that are less than several centimeters thick are often effectively treated using electrons. The depth of penetration of electrons is limited by their energy. This is an advantage because normal tissues deep to a tumor can be spared from receiving excessive radiation dose by careful selection of the electron energy. Linear accelerators usually have a range of electron energies available that can treat tumors up to 4 to 6 cm thick and the radiation oncologist can perform manual calculations to determine the machine settings for radiation delivery. As electrons have a mass and a charge, they are easily scattered by interactions with air molecules between the linear accelerator and the patient so special electron cones or applicators (**Fig. 1**) are used to shape the treatment field and assure uniformity of the electron beam. For periocular treatment fields, paraffin-coated lead contacts can be used to shield the eye from unwanted radiation dose.

2D Photon Therapy

This technique of radiation delivery uses one or more beams of photons directed at the tumor. A typical beam orientation would involve parallel-opposed beams centered on the tumor. A collimator in the linear accelerator is used to crudely shape the treatment fields, typically square or rectangular, to include the tumor and avoid the inclusion of excessive volumes of normal tissue. Unlike electrons, photons have no mass and no charge and penetrate into the patient to treat deeper tumors. Like electron therapy, the radiation oncologist performs manual calculations to determine the machine settings

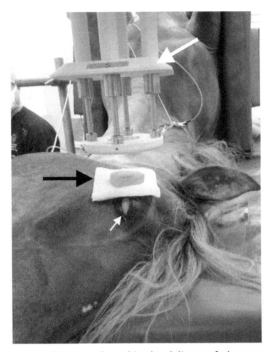

Fig. 1. An electron cone (*white arrow*) used in the delivery of electron radiation to a periocular sarcoid. Wet gauze and bolus material (*black arrow*) are used to assure appropriate radiation dose to the tumor. Note the paraffin-coated lead contact shielding the eye (*yellow arrow*).

for radiation delivery. Also, like electron therapy, this technique is simple and can be performed relatively easily.

3D Photon Therapy

This technique is used when it is critically important to limit side effects to normal tissues around the tumor. It requires a CT image of the patient positioned as they would be for treatment in a positioning mattress that is used by the radiation oncologist to design a more complicated treatment plan. The plan is created using a treatment planning software and often consists of multiple beams of radiation more precisely shaped to irradiate the tumor while strategically sparing normal tissue. A CT or radiographs are performed using the linear accelerator prior to each treatment to assure accurate patient positioning and appropriate radiation dose delivery as patient malpositioning will result in underdosing the tumor and overdosing normal tissues, leading to poor tumor control and unnecessary side effects. This technique cannot be performed on horses without some modification to a typical linear accelerator due to interference between the built-in couch, gantry, and the hydraulic table supporting the horse.

TELETHERAPY RADIATION PROTOCOLS

The dose of radiation delivered is measured in the International Unit of the Gray (Gy), which is the amount of radiation absorbed in a mass of tissue. Radiation protocols are designed to deliver a total dose of radiation in a predetermined number of smaller individual doses, termed fractions. Each fraction is delivered daily, every other day, or weekly depending on the intent of the treatment. Radiation protocols are typically termed either definitive or palliative in intent. Definitive-intent protocols typically involve numerous daily or every other day fractions of small doses of radiation for several weeks resulting in high total doses. Palliative-intent protocols involve fewer, larger fractions delivered every other day or once weekly resulting in lower total doses. Because of the fewer number of fractions in palliative protocols, they are often referred to as coarse fractioned as there are some tumor types that have demonstrated a better response to such a protocol and palliation is not necessarily the goal of the therapy. The decision to pursue a given protocol is determined by considering several factors: the expected response of the tumor to radiation, if known; the severity of anticipated side effects to the normal tissues in the region; the safety of repeated general anesthesia; and the owner's goals.

SIDE EFFECTS OF RADIOTHERAPY

The side effects of radiotherapy are the consequence of the death of normal cells in the treated area around the tumor and can be categorized as acute or late based on when they are expected to occur. Acute side effects occur near the end or after the conclusion of the radiotherapy and are a consequence of the death of rapidly dividing normal cells, typically those in epithelial tissue like skin or mucous membranes, resulting in dermatitis or mucositis. Higher total radiation doses are more likely to result in acute side effects. Because epithelial tissues have a stem-cell population, the tissue heals with time. Late effects can occur in any tissue and are typically the consequence of the death of slowly dividing cells like vascular and lymphatic endothelium. Dermal fibrosis and leukotrichia can be seen following irradiation of cutaneous tumors (**Fig. 2**). Frequently, these side effects are cosmetic and pose no clinical problems. In rare cases, with excessive dose to skin or bone, loss of vascularity in the tissues occurs, resulting in nonhealing cutaneous wounds or osteoradionecrosis. Once these side effects begin, there is nothing that can be done to stop the progression, and treatment focuses on management of the wound and any clinical signs. These side effects can be very problematic and may necessitate surgical correction, when possible.

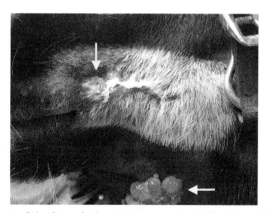

Fig. 2. Lateral aspect of the face of a horse (nose is to the left) showing leukotrichia in the treated radiation field around a scar from a previous sarcoid resection. The sarcoid had recurred along the rostral end of the scar, prompting radiation treatment. The tumor has regressed (*yellow arrow*) in response to the treatment. The patient subsequently developed another sarcoid (*white arrow*) outside the radiation field several weeks after the treatment.

SPECIAL CONSIDERATIONS FOR EQUINE RADIOTHERAPY

Because of their size, horses cannot be positioned on a traditional linear accelerator couch. At the authors' institution, horses are placed in dorsal recumbency on a hydraulic surgery table. The linear accelerator couch is rotated to the side, allowing the hydraulic table to get close enough to position the treated area in the beam path (**Fig. 3**). The area to be irradiated must be positioned at the isocenter of the machine. Due to the size of the horse and hydraulic table, radiation therapy is limited to the head and cranial neck, and limbs from the carpus and tarsus distally at the authors' institution. Most radiotherapy facilities cannot treat horses due to the limitation of access to the inside of the linear accelerator vault. At the authors' institution, the vault was designed with a lead door large enough for a horse on a hydraulic table to pass through, built into the side of the maze. The vault must also be large enough to accommodate the anesthetic machine and any monitoring equipment necessary. At the authors' institution, a camera allows the patient and machine to be seen during treatment and the patient's parameters (electrocardiogram, pulse oximetry, end tidal CO_2) are displayed on a monitor at the treatment console outside the vault.

Because the horse is positioned in dorsal recumbency at our institution, the head and neck must be rotated into lateral to treat lesions on the dorsal surface as the gantry cannot be rotated under the hydraulic table. Limbs must be extended and held using ropes tied to the table to allow the treated area to be positioned in the beam path and allow the gantry to rotate around the limb (**Fig. 4**).

REPORTS OF RADIATION THERAPY IN HORSES: WHAT IS THE EVIDENCE?

Sarcoids are the tumor type most commonly reported to be treated with radiation, with the majority treated with brachytherapy.[2–7] Good outcomes have been reported for treatment of periocular and nonocular sarcoids with high dose rate brachytherapy (**Table 1**). Literature describing the treatment of sarcoids using teletherapy is limited but has been performed for 21 years at the authors' institution.[8] Teletherapy has been used to treat 49 sarcoids at the authors' institution, the majority being periocular. There was recurrence in 8 cases, although follow up was limited in many cases (unpublished

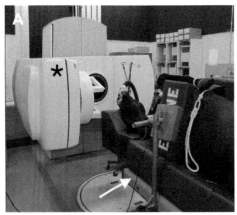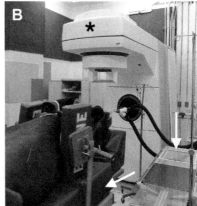

Fig. 3. A horse positioned on a hydraulic table (*white arrows*) and positioned for the treatment of a tumor in the rostral mandible. (*A*) The gantry (*asterisk*) is rotated to 270°. (*B*) The gantry (*asterisk*) is rotated to 0° and the linear accelerator couch (*yellow arrow*) is positioned to the side to allow the hydraulic table access to the radiation beam path.

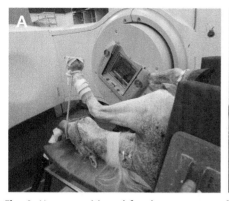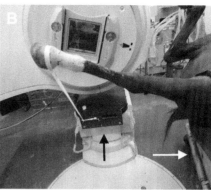

Fig. 4. Horses positioned for the treatment of a forelimb (*A*) and a hindlimb (*B*). Both patients were treated with photons using parallel-opposed beams with the gantry positioned at 90° (shown in both). The limbs are extended and restrained with rope or tape. The area around the limb is kept clear to allow rotation of the gantry around the limb. Note the linear accelerator couch rotated to 90° (*B, black arrow*) and hydraulic table (*B, white arrow*).

data). Side effects have included self-limiting ocular irritation, 3 cases of mild desquamation, and 2 cases with skin necrosis.

Ocular squamous cell carcinoma (SCC) in horses has been reported to have a lower reoccurrence rate when treated with radiation, whether teletherapy, brachytherapy, or plesiotherapy.[10] Recurrence has been reported in 12% to 17% of ocular/periocular SCC cases treated with adjunctive radiation therapy, compared to 44% recurrence without radiation therapy (see **Table 1**).[10–12] It is important to note that the majority of cases reported in the literature received surgical excision or debulking in addition to radiation therapy, and some received local chemotherapy or cryotherapy as well. The location, tumor depth, and availability of radiation equipment will determine which type of radiation treatment is most appropriate. Although SCC tends to be locally invasive, it also has the potential to metastasize, so careful evaluation of regional lymph nodes is recommended prior to starting a course of radiation therapy.

Nasal and paranasal sinus tumors are challenging to treat since their location often prevents surgical excision with large margins. Teletherapy with photons is the treatment of choice in this region due to the deeper penetration. Although reported case numbers are low, response to radiation appears to be good for horses with lymphoma and ossifying fibroma and guarded in horses with SCC (see **Table 1**).[14–20] Survival after radiotherapy for horses with nasal and sinus tumors appears to be worse than for those with mandibular tumors, likely due to airway compromise and limited surgical access, but potentially also due to difficulties with accurate radiation dosing in this area or possibly inherent radioresistance of some of the tumors.[14]

Successful treatment with radiation has also been reported for horses with rhabdomyosarcoma, hamartoma, hemangioma, and malignant dermal schwannoma.[21–24] The authors have treated two Arabian horses with mast cell tumors of the distal limbs, one with partial response and one that had complete response with reoccurrence at 4 years. Radiation therapy of regional lymph nodes has been shown to improve survival in other species, for example, in dogs with high-grade mast cell tumor[25]; however, the impact of regional lymph node treatment on survival in horses is unknown. The authors have performed palliative treatment of regional mandibular lymph nodes in a horse with metastasis of SCC, with good response (decreased pain, swelling, and elimination of drainage) for approximately 10 months, but further metastasis at 12 months.

Table 1
Overview of published literature describing treatment of equine tumors using radiotherapy

References	Number of Horses	Tumor Type	Location	Modality	Side Effects	Outcome
Byam-Cook et al,[2] 2016	23	Sarcoid	Periocular (8) Nonocular (15)	Ir-192 interstitial brachytherapy	Mild leukotrichia, alopecia, and scar tissue in a few cases	CR in 8/8 periocular and 13/15 non-ocular 2 treatment failures were with fibroblastic sarcoids Follow up 4–91 mo
Hollis et al,[4] 2018	8	Sarcoid	Periocular	High dose rate brachytherapy		CR in 8/8 Follow up 10–12 mo
Hollis et al,[3] 2017	25	Sarcoid	Periocular	High dose rate brachytherapy	No significant adverse effects	96% CR
Knottenbelt and Kelly,[5] 2000	66	Sarcoid	Periocular	Interstitial brachytherapy		98% CR Follow up 6–12 mo
Walker et al,[6] 1991	12	Sarcoid	Eyelid (11) Neck (2), ear, face, tarsus	Ir-192 interstitial brachytherapy	Alopecia Necrosis (1)	87.5% CR ≥ 12 mo 81.2% CR ≥ 24 mo
Theon and Pascoe,[7] 1995	63 52	Sarcoid SCC	Periocular	Ir-192 interstitial brachytherapy		74% for sarcoids 63.5% for SCC Progression-free survival, 5 y follow up
Wyn-Jones,[9] 1983	26	Fibroma, fibropapillomata, myxofibroma, sarcoid, SCC	Periocular (21) Limbs (5)	Ir-192 interstitial brachytherapy	Alopecia, leukotrichia; Rare conjunctivitis‑	CR in all cases with follow up (# unknown) Follow up ≥ 12 mo
Mosunic et al,[10] 2004	91 (231 total treatments, 59 with adjuvant RT)	SCC	Ocular and adnexal	Brachytherapy (implants), strontium-90, teletherapy	Eyelid infection, blepharitis (2 in Ir-192 group)	Recurrence in 12% (vs 44% without radiation) Large % lost to follow up

Study	Number	Tumor type	Location	Radiation type	Adverse effects	Outcome
Plummer et al,[11] 2007	38	SCC	Corneolimbal	Strontium-90 (combined surgery)	None reported, other than recurrence	Reoccurrence in 17% Follow up > 1 y Mean tumor-free interval for those without reoccurrence = 57 mo
Walker et al,[12] 1986	17	SCC	Ocular and periocular	Strontium-90, interstitial brachytherapy	Dry skin, leukotrichia, hair loss, moist desquamation (1)	87.5% CR Follow up 2 y
Bradley et al,[13] 2017	3	Lymphoma, sarcoid, melanoma	Cutaneous sarcoid and melanoma, ocular lymphoma	Electronic brachytherapy	Skin fibrosis/scarring; continued growth of untreated melanomas	CR in all, 17–22 mo follow up
Theon,[8] 1998	27	SCC, osteoma, ameloblastoma, melanoma, myxosarcoma, lymphoma	Head (23) Extremity (4)	Teletherapy	Not reported	Local control 2–54 mo
Gillen et al,[14] 2020	32	Carcinoma, sarcoma, ossifying fibroma, lymphoma	Mandible, maxilla, nasal/paranasal sinuses	Teletherapy	Acute respiratory difficulty, corneal ulceration, trismus	38% CR overall Worse prognosis for nasal/paranasal tumors Follow up median 14 mo
Henson et al,[15] 2004	4	Lymphoma	Perineum, hock, nasal, maxilla	Teletherapy	Leukotrichia in 3; nasal septum perforation in 1; unilateral facial nerve paralysis in 1	100% CR Follow up 29–114 mo
Gerard et al,[16] 2010	1	Lymphoma	Nasal/paranasal	Teletherapy photons	Acute, temporary blindness	CR Follow up 2.5 y
Weaver et al,[17] 1996	1	Lymphoma	Intranasal and perineal	Teletherapy	Mild hair loss, leukotrichia	CR, follow up 1 y
Walker et al,[18] 1998	3	SCC	Paranasal sinuses	Teletherapy (Cobalt-60)	Alopecia, superficial skin necrosis, leukotrichia	PR in all 3 horses; metastasis in all 3 horses Follow up 31 mo - 6 y

Abbreviations: CR, complete remission, Ir-192, iridium 192, PR, partial remission; SCC, squamous cell carcinoma.

PATIENT MANAGEMENT

Whenever possible, skin tumors are removed with adequate margins and the tumor and margins are evaluated by histopathology to determine whether follow up treatment is required. If the surgical resection is determined to be incomplete or in cases of "high-risk" tumors (eg, invasive or poorly differentiated SCC), a variety of adjunctive treatments can be employed, including surgical revision, local chemotherapy (either implantable or electrochemotherapy), cryotherapy, and radiation therapy. For tumors where clean margins cannot be achieved, debulking may be performed prior to radiation to decrease the volume of tissue that needs to be treated. At the authors' institution, this approach is used with cutaneous sarcoids where the tumor is debulked so it is flush with the skin surface, and the first radiation treatment is delivered immediately after the debulking procedure. Owners should be warned of the risk of recurrence, and the possibility of the development of new tumors at distant locations, especially cutaneous tumors like sarcoids, melanomas, and SCCs.

It is important to determine what tissue will remain after the tumor is irradiated. There may be extensive skin loss or fibrosis if the tumor is large or deep. It is ideal to rebiopsy if the original biopsy is not recent, the biopsy results do not fit with the clinical picture, or the tumor has changed since the most recent biopsy. Horses with negative outcomes (tissue necrosis, reoccurrence) tend to have more extensive skin tumors with larger area and deeper tissue involvement. Although the authors do not routinely perform abdominal ultrasound and thoracic radiographs in every horse presenting for radiation therapy, the potential for regional lymph node metastasis should be considered carefully for tumor types such as SCC, with thorough palpation, ultrasound, and if needed, computed tomography and lymph node aspirate or biopsy to determine whether additional radiation treatment fields or other adjunctive therapy may be needed. Finally, when the horse's quality of life is poor and prognosis is guarded, euthanasia should be discussed with the owner, especially in cases where radiation therapy is unlikely to improve quality of life or survival time.

SUMMARY

There are a variety of options for the treatment of tumors in horses, and when radiation therapy is available, it should be considered when adequate tumor margins are difficult to achieve or the tumor type has a high rate of recurrence. There is evidence of good success rates for treatment of periocular sarcoids and SCC, with brachytherapy. Plesiotherapy, while limited to superficial tumors, has also been demonstrated to be an effective treatment for ocular and adnexal tumor SCC and sarcoids. Teletherapy allows treatment of superficial tumors with electrons and deeper tumors with photons, although based on configurations of the equipment, treatment is often limited to tumors of the head and distal extremities.

CLINICS CARE POINTS

- Teletherapy for equine patients requires specialized facilities to accommodate a large animal surgery table. Based on patient positioning relative to the beam path, treatment may be limited to the head, cranial neck, and distal limbs.
- Brachytherapy can be used to treat solid, accessible tumors. High dose rate brachytherapy allows treatment of horses without general anesthesia and without exposure of personnel to radiation.

- Plesiotherapy can be used to treat superficial tumors, ideally less than 1 cm diameter and 3 mm thickness, most often tumors of the eye and adnexal structures.
- Acute side effects include hair loss, dermatitis, and mucositis. Late side effects include cosmetic changes such as leukotrichia, and less commonly, skin or bone necrosis.
- Success rates for treatment of periocular sarcoids with brachytherapy have been reported at 74% to 98%. For ocular and adnexal SCC, remission after adjunctive radiation treatment ranges from 83% to 88%. There appears to be a guarded prognosis for horses with tumors of the nasal and paranasal sinuses treated with radiation, although horses with nasal lymphoma may have a good prognosis.

DISCLOSURE

The authors have nothing to disclose.

REFERENCES

1. Farrelly J, McEntee MC. A survey of veterinary radiation facilities in 2010. Vet Radiol Ultrasound 2014;55(6):638–43.
2. Byam-Cook KL, Henson FMD, Slater JD. Treatment of periocular and non-ocular sarcoids in 18 horses by interstitial brachytherapy with iridium-192. Vet Rec 2006; 159:337–41.
3. Hollis AR, Berlato D. High dose brachytherapy for the treatment of periorbital sarcoids in the horse. Equine Vet J 2017;49(Suppl 51):5–29.
4. Hollis AR, Berlato D. Initial experience with high dose rate brachytherapy of periorbital sarcoids in the horse. Equine Vet Educ 2018;30:444–9.
5. Knottenbelt DC, Kelly DF. The diagnosis and treatment of periorbital sarcoid in the horse: 445 cases from 1974 to 1999. Vet Ophthalmol 2000;3:169–91.
6. Walker M, Adams W, Hoskinson J, et al. Iridium-192 brachytherapy for equine sarcoid, one and two year remission rates. Vet Radiol 1991;32(4):206–8.
7. Théon AP, Pascoe JR. Iridium-192 interstitial brachytherapy for equine periocular tumors: treatment results and prognostic factors in 115 horses. Equine Vet J 1995;27:117–21.
8. Théon AP. Radiation therapy in the horse. Vet Clin North Amer Equine 1998;14(3): 673–88.
9. Wyn-Jones G. Treatment of equine cutaneous neoplasia by radiotherapy using iridium 192 linear sources. Equine Vet J 1983;15(4):361–5.
10. Mosunic CB, Moore PA, Carmichael KP, et al. Effects of treatment with and without adjuvant radiation therapy on recurrence of ocular and adnexal squamous cell carcinoma in horses: 157 cases (1985-2002). J Am Vet Med Assoc 2004;225:1733–8.
11. Plummer CE, Smith S, Andrew SE, et al. Combined keratectomy, strontium-90 irradiation, and permanent bulbar conjunctival grafts for corneolimbal squamous cell carcinomas in horses (1990-2002): 38 horses. Vet Ophthalmol 2007;10(1): 37–42.
12. Walker MA, Goble D, Geiser D. Two-year non-recurrence rates for equine ocular and periorbital squamous cell carcinoma following radiotherapy. Vet Radiol 1986; 27:146–8.
13. Bradley WM, Schilpp D, Khatibzedeh SM. Electronic brachytherapy used for the successful treatment of three different types of equine tumors. Equine Vet Educ 2017;29(6):293–8.

14. Gillen A, Mudge M, Caldwell F, et al. Outcome of external beam radiotherapy for treatment of noncutaneous tumors of the head in horses: 32 cases (1999-2015). J Vet Intern Med 2020;34:2808–16.
15. Henson FMD, Dixon K, Dobson JM. Treatment of 4 cases of equine lymphoma with megavoltage radiation. Equine Vet Educ 2004;16(6):312–4.
16. Gerard M, Pruitt A, Thrall DE. Radiation therapy communication: Nasal passage and paranasal sinus lymphoma in a pony. Vet Radiol Ultrasound 2010;51(1): 97–101.
17. Weaver MP, Dobson JM, Lane JG. Treatment of intranasal lymphoma in a horse by radiotherapy. Equine Vet J 1996;28(3):245–8.
18. Walker MA, Schumacher J, Schmitz DG, et al. Cobalt 60 radiotherapy for treatment of squamous cell carcinoma of the nasal cavity and paranasal sinuses in three horses. J Am Vet Med Assoc 1998;212(6):848–51.
19. Orsini JA, Baird DK, Ruggles AJ. Radiotherapy of a recurrent ossifying fibroma in the paranasal sinuses of a horse. J Am Vet Med Assoc 2004;224(9):1483–6.
20. Robbins SC, Arighi M, Ottewell G. The use of megavoltage radiation to treat juvenile mandibular ossifying fibroma in a horse. Can Vet J 1996;37:683–4.
21. Castleman WL, Toplon DE, Clark CK, et al. Rhabdomyosarcoma in 8 horses. Vet Pathol 2011;48(6):1144–50.
22. Conti F, Poujet L, Delverdier M, et al. High dose interstitial 192-Ir brachytherapy for the treatment of a recurrent dermal vascular hamartoma in a horse. Equine Vet Educ 2022;34(8):e337–43.
23. Kleiter M, Velde K, Hainsch E, et al. Radiation therapy communication: Equine hemangioma. Vet Radiol Ultrasound 2009;50(5):560–3.
24. Saulez MN, Voigt A, Steyl JCA, et al. Use of Ir192 interstitial brachytherapy for an equine malignant dermal schwannoma. Tydskr S Afr Vet 2009;80(4):264–9.
25. Mendez SE, Drobatz KJ, Duda LE, et al. Treating the locoregional lymph nodes with radiation and/or surgery significantly improves outcome in dogs with high-grade mast cell tumours. Vet Comp Oncol 2020;18(2):239–46.

What Is the Evidence Behind Sarcoid Treatments?

Anna R. Hollis, BVetMed, MSc (Clin Onc), SFHEA, FRCVS

KEYWORDS

- Equine • Tumor • Evidence-based • Sarcoid

KEY POINTS

- There is no single best treatment for sarcoids.
- Evidence for the majority of treatment options is lacking.
- Understanding the limitations of treatment enables appropriate selection of modalities according to the lesion type, location, horse, and owner circumstances.

SURGICAL EXCISION (INCLUDING DIODE LASER, CARBON DIOXIDE LASER, ELECTROSURGERY, AND CRYOSURGERY)

Sharp Surgical Excision

Sharp surgical excision has low success rates and risk of aggressive recurrence.[1] Success rates have been reported to be between 30% and 82%, with most recurrences seen within 6 months.[2–5] The wide discrepancy is likely to be at least partially due to technique, with wide excision and a "no touch" technique more likely to be successful. Margins of between 9 and 16 mm appear to be sufficient,[2,3,6] although other authors have suggested 2 to 3 cm margins.[4,7]

Surgical excision may be less useful for periocular sarcoids. When used to treat 28 periocular sarcoids, 82% recurred at or immediately adjacent to the surgical site.[1] Adjunctive treatments may also be considered alongside surgical excision, which may improve success rates following surgical intervention by treating any neoplastic cells remaining at the margins of excision.

Electrosurgery

Electrosurgery has a success rate of 86.8% when performed under general anesthesia and with a margin of at least 12 mm of apparently normal skin.[3] An electrosurgical instrument was used with a non-touch technique, gloves and instruments were changed following excision, and the wound was routinely closed after rinsing with a chlorhexidine solution. The addition of cisplatin beads was associated with reduced success

Department of Veterinary Medicine, University of Cambridge, Madingley Road, Cambridge CB3 0ES, UK
E-mail address: arh207@cam.ac.uk

Vet Clin Equine 40 (2024) 409–419
https://doi.org/10.1016/j.cveq.2024.07.006
vetequine.theclinics.com
0749-0739/24/© 2024 Elsevier Inc. All rights reserved, including those for text and data mining, AI training, and similar technologies.

rates.[3] This is hard to explain but could be due to differences in case selection, if cisplatin beads were used in cases where margins were less clear and therefore less likely to be successfully treated. Regardless, electrosurgery appears to be a useful sole treatment of sarcoids in the hands of a skilled surgeon.

Laser Surgical Excision

Successful treatment of 83% of sarcoids has been reported with diode laser surgical excision.[8] Higher recurrence rates were observed when lesions were verrucose in any location, and when any form of sarcoid was located on the head and neck.[8] Limited skin mobility and the close approximation of sensitive tissues may make lesions on the head and neck more difficult to excise with wide margins. Verrucose sarcoids may have a less defined margin, which may make successful surgical treatment less likely unless a very wide margin of visually "normal" tissue is also removed. In contrast, carbon dioxide laser surgery has a success rate of 62% to 66.7%.[7,9] Diode laser excision leads to a wider zone of damage, which may be more likely to achieve clean "margins" and therefore lead to a higher chance of success.

The major downside to any form of laser surgical excision is the prolonged healing time. Some surgeons close the tissue where feasible, but many lesions are left to heal by secondary intention. Horses generally show minimal signs of pain following laser surgery. This makes laser excision a practical first-line treatment for most sarcoid lesions.

Cryosurgery

When performed following surgical debulking of saroids, cryosurgery has reported success rates of 70% to 80%.[2,10,11] This usually involves the application of liquid nitrogen via a spray or probe at $-196°C$ to the area in question. Both nitrous oxide and carbon dioxide systems are available. Inconsistent temperatures have been demonstrated with both gases, related to the devices used rather than the gas itself.[12] The extremely cold temperature leads to the formation of intracellular ice and cell membrane rupture, destroying tumor tissue. Thermocouples should be used to monitor the temperature and depth of the freeze, with 3 freeze–thaw cycles decreasing the tissue temperature to -20 to $-30°C$ recommended,[13] to include a margin of normal tissue surrounding the visible lesion. The tissue sloughs 2 to 4 weeks later, and depigmentation may persist. Repeated treatments may be required, and severe contraction of the surgical scar is a potential complication.

One report suggests that cryosurgery may be inappropriate for the treatment of periocular sarcoids. In 28 cases, 91% had aggressive recurrence within 12 weeks, and in some cases, uncontrollable disease led to euthanasia.[1]

TOPICAL TREATMENTS

Many topical creams are available for the treatment of sarcoids, with various protocols and success rates, and limited published data. In general, topical formulations are simple and convenient to use and are often relatively low cost.

The use of topical creams for the treatment of periocular sarcoids is complicated by the proximity to the globe and the potential for severe collateral damage.[14] In this location, topical creams may only be useful in the treatment of small, superficial lesions (deep margins measuring <5 mm).[15]

There is a risk of the material spreading to the skin around the lesion ("run off") in any location, which is almost impossible to prevent even with meticulous application. Many of these substances are irritants, so the horse may also rub the site, spreading the material to untreated areas. Spread will cause unwanted, secondary damage and can reduce efficacy at the treated site, as some of the material has been lost. Handler exposure is a risk and should not be underestimated; accidental exposure to chemo-therapeutic compounds is a potentially significant health and safety issue.

Topical application leads to uncertain intralesional distribution within the tumor. Repeated applications are often necessary, and many treatments may only be useful for superficial tumors. Anecdotally, removing heavily keratinized tissue in the case of verrucose sarcoids (eg, using retinoid creams prior to chemotherapy compounds, or via debridement of the abnormal tissue) may increase the likelihood of successful treatment.

Topical materials can also cause an uncontrolled response to treatment. This may lead to treatment failure and the need to repeat the treatment course, or to a very strong response to treatment leading to a poor cosmetic or functional outcome. The use of topical creams in areas where function is potentially impeded by scar tissue (eg, periocular lesions and those around the lip commissure) is, therefore, not gener-ally recommended.

5-Fluorouracil

5-Fluorouracil (5-FU) is a readily available topical treatment that has been reported to be successful in around 67% of superficial lesions around the eye,[1] but more recently, a success rate of only 26.7% was seen in a small number of lesions treated with a pro-tocol of twice a day application for 10 days.[16] When this protocol of topical 5-FU was combined with a follow-up treatment using ultra-deformable bleomycin-containing li-posomes, the success rate increased to 77%, far greater than the success rate when the bleomycin was used a sole treatment.[16] It is hard to know why there is such a discrepancy in the success rates, but the author has used this clinically to good effect in superficial lesions.

AW Formulations

A compounded chemotherapy-based cream, AW3, AW4, and more recently AW5, is commonly used to treat sarcoids in the United Kingdom, despite limited published data. One publication has suggested that a success rate of over 80% was achieved with the application of AW3, but no details of the treatment protocol, type of sarcoids, or other clinical features were presented.[17] A success rate of 35% has been reported for AW3 in a small number of periocular sarcoids.[1] To the author's knowledge, details of the ingredients, protocol, utility, and success rate of AW cream for sarcoid lesions have not been published in a peer-reviewed publication, but anecdotally this appears to be a successful treatment for many lesions.

The main limiting factor is that the preparation requires multiple applications, which must be performed by a veterinary surgeon. Following treatment, marked swelling is expected and horses often become very painful. The treated lesion will eventually form an eschar that sloughs off, leaving a large area that will heal via secondary inten-tion if no sarcoid tissue remains. Lesions at the lip commissure and on the upper eyelid are prone to significant scar contracture, leading to deformities and functional is-sues,[17] and a fatality following erosion through the abdominal wall and subsequent evisceration has been reported.[18]

Although the exact composition is unknown, the formulation contains a variety of toxic substances that have health and safety implications for those handling the horse. These risks should not be understated to those whose horses are receiving this treatment.

Imiquimod

Imiquimod is an immune modifier sometimes used for the treatment of superficial sarcoids, requiring application 3 times a week until clinical resolution. Treatment can be performed by the owner, but horses typically become challenging to treat because of the associated discomfort. Feeding the horse during application of the cream may help with the process. It has been recommended that prior to each application, the treated area is gently cleaned, and it is this process that the horses appear to resent the most — but it is likely to be critical to ensure penetration of the cream. It is important to emphasize the importance of personal safety where owners use this treatment (such as applying imiquimod wearing gloves and avoiding handling the treated area). A response rate of 60% to 84.4% for small, superficial lesions has been reported, with treatment duration ranging from 4 to 45 weeks.[3,19,20] A small retrospective case series found that combination of imiquimod with tazarotene had a reported efficacy of "up to 100%,"[21] so the combination of these 2 treatments may also be useful.

Bloodroot Ointment (Sanguinaria canadensis)

Bloodroot plant extracts (Sanguinaria canadensis) have been used for sarcoid treatment, with 58% of lesions in any location resolving following treatment with the ointment in an owner-based survey.[22] The protocol varied from 1 to greater than 42 days, so it is hard to make definitive recommendations, but it appears that it may be useful in some cases. A more recent study looked at the use of a combination of S canadensis with zinc chloride, available as a commercial preparation (Xxterra), where 75% of tumors responded — but it is important to note that of these, 21.4% of lesions relapsed,[20] so an overall success rate of 53.6% appears to be more accurate. The treatment duration varied from 4 to 38 weeks, and inclusion criteria were lacking,[20] so further work is needed.

Acyclovir

Acyclovir is a controversial treatment. A success rate of 53% to 68% in small, early sarcoid lesions has been reported,[3,23] although confusingly acyclovir has also been associated with treatment failures.[3] A placebo-controlled study of acyclovir treatment of occult and verrucose sarcoids failed to show any advantage over placebo.[24]

The potential mechanism of action of acyclovir in equine sarcoids is questionable. Acyclovir is marketed to treat human herpesvirus-induced skin lesions, and its antiviral properties are only active following triple phosphorylation by viral and cellular thymidine kinases.[25] Papillomaviruses lack the gene coding for viral thymidine kinase and are therefore cannot activate acyclovir. However, there was an increased antiproliferative effect of acyclovir in bovine papillomavirus infected compared to virus-free equine fibroblastic cell lines, suggesting interaction of acyclovir with bovine papillomavirus (BPV)-infected cells.[23] It is possible that cellular tyrosine kinases may activate the antiviral effect of acyclovir, but this has not been proven. Acyclovir is simple and safe for owners to apply and is readily available as a human "over-the-counter" cold sore ointment. More data are required to fully evaluate its place in equine sarcoid treatment.

Topical Bleomycin

In general, bleomycin has poor penetration. Ultra-deformable liposomes containing bleomycin have been formulated, and in carefully selected cases, bleomycin with 5-FU or tazarotene was more effective than either treatment alone.[16] Skin irritation and soreness appear inevitable, despite initial reports that horses are not painful with the treatment.[16] There is limited evidence for this treatment and more data are required, especially as the current protocols involve extended treatment periods and are expensive.

Tazarotene

Tazarotene is a retinoid cream with a success rate of 17.1% when used alone, although combined with bleomycin this increased to 77.8%, an improvement to the success rate of bleomycin alone.[16] Tazarotene appears to be most useful prior to other topical treatments, presumably because it improves penetration of other substances.

Betulinic Acid

Betulinic acid is extracted from the bark of the white birch, permeates equine skin in vitro, and has anticancer activity against equine fibroblastic cells.[26] When applied topically to the skin of healthy horses, it was well tolerated, with only mild local adverse effects.[27] To date, to this author's knowledge, it has not been used clinically for sarcoids but it may yet reach clinical use if in vitro translates to in vivo utility.

INTRALESIONAL CHEMOTHERAPY

There are limited published data on the success rate of intralesional chemotherapy other than intralesional cisplatin, and there are significant health and safety implications.

Intralesional Cisplatin

Injectable forms of cisplatin

A 96% success rate has been reported in a large number of sarcoids following intralesional cisplatin.[28] These results have not been replicated in other studies and probably reflect careful case selection. In particular, accurate injection of cisplatin can be difficult and was successful in only 33% of periocular sarcoid cases,[1] and in other locations, the success rate has been reported to be 53%.[3] Intralesional platinum-based chemotherapy drugs have also been associated with treatment failure.[3] It is difficult to make specific recommendations for its use, especially given the potential for exposure of the operator and handlers of the horse to chemotherapeutic agents.

Cisplatin beads

Intralesional cisplatin beads may be useful, with 91% of lesions showing long-term resolution in one small study of 22 cases over a 2 year time period. The side effects were minor, including alopecia, swelling, and scarring.[29] The improved health and safety profile of cisplatin beads over intralesional injections of liquid cisplatin is enticing—they are easier to handle, there are no concerns with the difficulty of injecting material into firm sarcoid tissue, and the frequency of treatment is reduced.[13] The potential for exposure to cisplatin residues remains.

Intralesional Mitomycin C

There are limited data around the use of intralesional mitomycin C. A very small number of periocular sarcoid cases have been reported with limited follow-up.[30] Anecdotally, it is the author's experience that this may be successful for nodular and fibroblastic lesions, but it has also led to widespread skin necrosis and treatment failures.

Intralesional 5-Flourouracil

In a small case series, intralesional 5-FU has been reported to have a long-term success rate of 61.5%.[31] It may therefore be useful for the treatment of some lesions.

Other Intralesional Medications

Carboplatin and bleomycin may also be used intralesionally. Intralesional carboplatin was associated with treatment failures and was inferior to electrosurgery in one study.[3] To the author's knowledge, there are no peer-reviewed published data on the use of intralesional bleomycin.

Tigilanol tiglate is a novel compound licensed to treat canine mast cell tumors. Its "tumor agnostic" mode of action leads to an acute inflammatory response with immune cell recruitment and disruption of tumor vasculature. It has been reported to be successful in a single periocular sarcoid,[32] and the author has used it in a small number of cases with good results (Hollis 2024, unpublished data). Intralesional injection leads to rapid hemorrhagic necrosis of the tumor and a subsequent slough of the necrotic tumor mass, followed by infill of the tissue defect and re-epithelization of the treatment site, with good functional outcomes.[32] Although this is a very interesting novel treatment, the current lack of meaningful data makes specific recommendations impossible.

ALVAC-fIL2, a feline interleukin-2 immunomodulator commercially available as Oncept IL-2, has also been used as an intralesional treatment of a small number of sarcoids.[33] Seven of 14 lesions regressed, and a further 5 had a partial response.[33] This is worthy of further investigation, although it is very expensive that will limit its utility compared to other options.

ELECTROCHEMOTHERAPY

Electrochemotherapy has a reported success rate of 94% to 100% in a large number of cases.[34–36] General anesthesia is a prerequisite for treatment and larger lesions require several treatments. However, disadvantages of general anesthesia aside, its impressive success rates in a reasonable number of cases mean that it is worthy of consideration. Lesions are injected with a chemotherapeutic compound (generally cisplatin), and electrochemotherapy is used to increase the penetration into the cells. The use of cisplatin is associated with significant health and safety concerns during and after administration. Personnel handling the horse following treatment should wear appropriate personal protective equipment.

PHOTODYNAMIC THERAPY

Photodynamic therapy requires a photodynamic substance to be applied to the sarcoid, followed (some hours later) by the application of light of a specific wavelength according to the photodynamic substance used. Most photodynamic substances have poor penetration, making the technique only suitable for superficial lesions or as an adjunctive therapy. When used with a penetration enhancer, response rates improved from 14% to 93%,[37] although there was only 1 month of follow-up, limiting its utility as a study as sarcoid recurrences are usually over a longer time frame. Photodynamic therapy is unlikely to be a useful sole treatment, but it may be a useful adjunctive therapy alongside laser or sharp surgical excision. The application of photodynamic therapy is a prolonged process; the photodynamic substance must be left in situ for several hours without being exposed to light prior to the treatment. In addition, the treatment appears to be painful, with most horses requiring sedation.

IMMUNOTHERAPY
Bacillus Calmette and Guerin and Mycobacterium Cell Wall Extracts

Bacillus Calmette and Guerin (BCG) is an attenuated strain of Mycobacterium bovis. When injected intra-tumourally, BCG is believed to stimulate local cell-mediated immune responses, inducing natural killer and cytotoxic T cells that eliminate tumor cells.[38,39]

Intralesional BCG has a success rate of 58% to 69% when used for nodular and fibroblastic periocular lesions but appears to be unsuccessful when used in verrucose and occult lesions, as well as when used in other locations.[1,3] Anaphylaxis appears relatively unusual, especially when the treatment is combined with premedication with nonsteroidal anti-inflammatory drugs and/or dexamethasone. BCG is difficult to obtain, but Mycobacterium cell wall extracts are readily available. One locally injected Mycobacterium cell wall fraction had a 52.9% complete resolution rate, and a further 17.6% had improved but not resolved at the time of follow-up.[40] Intralesional injections are repeated every 2 to 4 weeks until regression, averaging 3 treatments.[41] The success rate of BCG in lesions in locations other than around the eye is lower, with success rates of around 50% reported in the literature,[4,42–44] consistent with the reported success rate of the commercially available Mycobacterium cell wall extract in a variety of locations.[40]

RADIOTHERAPY

Radiotherapy is considered the "gold standard" for periocular sarcoids,[1,14,16,45] but its high cost and limited availability are significant barriers. Periocular sarcoids have been treated with low-dose brachytherapy for over 40 years, but the availability of this modality has become increasingly limited because of the high cost of the sources, health and safety concerns, and practicalities around their use.[45] High-dose rate brachytherapy eliminates operator exposure and many of the health and safety concerns, although this technique remains expensive and extremely limited in availability.[45] Unlike low-dose rate techniques, high-dose rate brachytherapy does not require isolation of the horse—treatments can be performed under standing sedation and the treatment times are very short.

Strontium plesiotherapy is a locally applied, superficial form of radiotherapy described for the treatment of sarcoids.[1,46] It appears to be very effective. However, it is only suitable for use in the treatment of very small, superficial lesions due to its limited penetration. It is simple, cost-effective, does not require isolation of the horse, and usually requires only standing sedation, but it has very limited availability.

Teletherapy has also been used for equine sarcoids.[47] This is radiotherapy delivered via a linear accelerator, requiring multiple general anesthetics over several days to weeks. This is rarely accessible due to the limited availability and high cost of treatment.

Electronic brachytherapy has successfully treated a single sarcoid.[48] The technique requires multiple general anesthetics and could be used as a sole treatment or combined with other modalities. There are no published data on its efficacy in any other lesions in any other location, and no longer term follow-up is available of this single case.

SYSTEMIC TREATMENT OPTIONS
Autologous Vaccination

Autologous vaccination is a potential treatment option for equine sarcoids. One report found a 100% success rate,[49] with another trial finding that although 24% of cases developed recurrences following autologous vaccination, remission was achieved in 80% of these following repeat treatment.[50] A study of 18 horses treated via this method found that owner-reported clinical regression was observed in 69% and a reduction in the number of sarcoids in 75% of cases.[51] Autologous vaccination has failed to find widespread favor, possibly because there are also reports of aggressive regrowth of sarcoids at implantation sites.[52]

Mistletoe Extract (Viscum Album Austriacus)

A placebo-controlled study of the use of mistletoe extract (*viscum album austriacus*) investigated subcutaneous administration in increasing concentrations 3 times a week over 105 days. Complete regression was observed in 38% of lesions with few side effects.[53] While the overall success of this treatment is low, the ease of administration makes it a potentially interesting option in horses with many lesions.

Intravenous Doxorubicin

One report suggested that intravenous doxorubicin may be potentially useful for sarcoids.[54] It appeared to be active against fast-growing, fibroblastic sarcoids, but less active against slow-growing, verrucose lesions; the overall response rate was likely to be between 10% and 50% based on a small number of treated lesions.[54] Given the large number of other potentially effective sarcoid treatments and the logistical difficulties, cost, and potential side effects of administering intravenous doxorubicin to horses, it seems unlikely that this treatment will become a routine treatment of horses, but it could be considered in end-stage cases.

Is There Any Truly Evidence-Based Treatment Strategy for Sarcoids?

It is this author's belief that, based on the limited evidence base, appropriate treatment options vary with the location and type of the sarcoid, and no one treatment is universally appropriate.[55] Numerous options are available, varying with the location and type of sarcoid, treatment accessibility, and financial constraints. Many are expensive and time-consuming, and some have additional health and safety implications. It is therefore vital to take all the relevant patient, owner, and lesion factors into account to make the best possible decision for the case in question. A recent systematic review was performed investigating the evidence for the selection of sarcoid treatment and concluded that there was insufficient evidence available to recommend any specific treatment over another.[56] It is clear that large, multicenter, international clinical trials investigating the available treatment options are required to truly understand the utility of the myriad of treatment options. The logistics around this approach make it sadly unlikely to ever be performed.

CLINICS CARE POINTS

- There is no one universally applicable treatment for all sarcoids. Treatment selection should be based on the lesion type, location, owner preferences, and availability of the treatment.
- Based on the current evidence, laser surgical resection is the most appropriate first-line treatment in the majority of cases due to its high success rates and ease of availability.

DISCLOSURE

The author has no affiliations other than I work for the University of Cambridge.

REFERENCES

1. Knottenbelt DC, Kelly DF. The diagnosis and treatment of periorbital sarcoid in the horse: 445 cases from 1974 to 1999. Vet Ophthalmol 2000;3:169–91.
2. Martens A, De Moor A, Vlaminck L, et al. Evaluation of excision, cryosurgery and local BCG vaccination for the treatment of equine sarcoids. Vet Rec 2001;149: 665–9.
3. Haspeslagh M, Vlaminck LE, Martens AM. Treatment of sarcoids in equids: 230 cases (2008-2013). J Am Vet Med Assoc 2016;249:311–8.
4. McConaghy FF, Davis RE, Reppas GP, et al. Management of equine sarcoids: 1975-1993. N Z Vet J 1994;42:180–4.
5. Genetzky RM, Biwer RD, Myers RK. Equine sarcoids, causes, diagnosis, and treatment. Compend Continuing Educ Pract Vet 1983;5:S416.
6. Martens A, De Moor A, Demeulemeester J, et al. Polymerase chain reaction analysis of the surgical margins of equine sarcoids for bovine papilloma virus DNA. Vet Surg 2001;30:460–7.
7. Carstanjen B, Jordan P, Lepage OM. Carbon dioxide laser as a surgical instrument for sarcoid therapy–a retrospective study on 60 cases. Can Vet J 1997; 38:773–6.
8. Compston PC, Turner T, Wylie CE, et al. Laser surgery as a treatment for histologically confirmed sarcoids in the horse. Equine Vet J 2016;48:451–6.
9. McCauley CT, Hawkins JF, Adams SB, et al. Use of a carbon dioxide laser for surgical management of cutaneous masses in horses: 32 cases (1993-2000). J Am Vet Med Assoc 2002;220:1192–7.
10. Lane JG. The treatment of equine sarcoids by cryosurgery. Equine Vet J 1977;9: 127–33.
11. Fretz PB, Barber SM. Prospective analysis of cryosurgery as the sole treatment for equine sarcoids. Vet Clin N Am Equine Pract 1980;10:847–59.
12. Winkler JL, Jeronimo J, Singleton J, et al. Performance of cryotherapy devices using nitrous oxide and carbon dioxide. Int J Gynaecol Obstet 2010;111:73–7.
13. Hewes CA, Sullins KE. Review of the treatment of equine cutaneous neoplasia. AAEP proceedings 2009;55:386–93.
14. Hollis AR. Radiotherapy for the treatment of periocular tumours in the horse. Equine Vet Educ 2019;31:647–52.
15. Malalana F. Treatment of periocular tumours - what is the evidence? BEVA congress 2015;66.
16. Knottenbelt DC, Watson AH, Hotchkiss JW, et al. A pilot study on the use of ultradeformable liposomes containing bleomycin in the treatment of equine sarcoid. Equine Vet Educ 2018;32:258–63.
17. Knottenbelt DC, Walker JA. Topical treatment of the equine sarcoid. Equine Vet Educ 1994;6:72–5.
18. Baldwin AJ, Mair TS, Busschers E. Evisceration in a Thoroughbred gelding following application of a topical chemotherapy agent for the treatment of sarcoids. Equine Vet Educ 2023;35:e475–8.
19. Nogueira SA, Torres SM, Malone ED, et al. Efficacy of imiquimod 5% cream in the treatment of equine sarcoids: a pilot study. Vet Dermatol 2006;17:259–65.
20. Pettersson CM, Brostrom H, Humblot P, et al. Topical treatment of equine sarcoids with imiquimod 5% cream or Sanguinaria canadensis and zinc chloride - an open prospective study. Vet Dermatol 2020;31:471-e126.

21. Tamzali Y, Boidot m. Use of combination of tazarotene cream and imiquimod 5% cream in the treatment of equine sarcoids: a 20 case retrospective study. J Vet Intern Med 2014;28:709.

22. Wilford S, Woodward B, Dunkel B. Efficacy of bloodroot ointment for the treatment of equine sarcoids. J Vet Intern Med 2013;28:704.

23. Stadler S, Kainzbauer C, Haralambus R, et al. Successful treatment of equine sarcoids by topical aciclovir application. Vet Rec 2011;168:187.

24. Haspeslagh M, Jordana Garcia M, Vlaminck LEM, et al. Topical use of 5% acyclovir cream for the treatment of occult and verrucous equine sarcoids: a double-blinded placebo-controlled study. BMC Vet Res 2017;13:296.

25. Elion GB. The biochemistry and mechanism of action of acyclovir. J Antimicrob Chemother 1983;12(Suppl B):9–17.

26. Weber LA, Meissner J, Delarocque J, et al. Betulinic acid shows anticancer activity against equine melanoma cells and permeates isolated equine skin in vitro. BMC Vet Res 2020;16:44.

27. Weber LA, Puff C, Kalbitz J, et al. Concentration profiles and safety of topically applied betulinic acid and NVX-207 in eight healthy horses-A randomized, blinded, placebo-controlled, crossover pilot study. J Vet Pharmacol Therapeut 2021;44:47–57.

28. Theon AP, Wilson WD, Magdesian KG, et al. Long-term outcome associated with intratumoral chemotherapy with cisplatin for cutaneous tumors in equidae: 573 cases (1995-2004). J Am Vet Med Assoc 2007;230:1506–13.

29. Hewes CA, Sullins KE. Use of cisplatin-containing biodegradable beads for treatment of cutaneous neoplasia in equidae: 59 cases (2000-2004). J Am Vet Med Assoc 2006;229:1617–22.

30. McKane SA. A practical protocol for the clinical use of mitomycin C in the treatment of sarcoids in horses. J Vet Intern Med 2014;28:704.

31. Stewart AA, Rush B, Davis E. The efficacy of intratumoural 5-fluorouracil for the treatment of equine sarcoids. Aust Vet J 2006;84:101–6.

32. De Ridder T, Ruppin M, Wheeless M, et al. Use of the Intratumoural Anticancer Drug Tigilanol Tiglate in Two Horses. Front Vet Sci 2020;7:639.

33. Saba C, Eggleston R, Parks A, et al. ALVAC-fIL2, a feline interleukin-2 immunomodulator, as a treatment for sarcoids in horses: A pilot study. J Vet Intern Med 2022;36:1179–84.

34. Tozon N, Kramaric P, Kos Kadunc V, et al. Electrochemotherapy as a single or adjuvant treatment to surgery of cutaneous sarcoid tumours in horses: a 31-case retrospective study. Vet Rec 2016;179:627.

35. Rols MP, Tamzali Y, Teissie J. Electrochemotherapy of horses. A preliminary clinical report. Bioelectrochemistry 2002;55:101–5.

36. Tamzali Y, Borde L, Rols MP, et al. Successful treatment of equine sarcoids with cisplatin electrochemotherapy: a retrospective study of 48 cases. Equine Vet J 2012;44:214–20.

37. Golding JP, Kemp-Symonds JG, Dobson JM. Glycolysis inhibition improves photodynamic therapy response rates for equine sarcoids. Vet Comp Oncol 2017;15:1543–52.

38. Davies M. Bacillus Calmette-Guerin as an anti-tumor agent. The interaction with cells of the mammalian immune system. Biochim Biophys Acta 1982;651:143–74.

39. Misdorp W, Klein WR, Ruitenberg EJ, et al. Clinico-pathological aspects of immunotherapy by intralesional injection of BCG cell walls or live BCG in bovine ocular squamous cell carcinoma. Cancer Immunol Immunother 1985;20:223–30.

40. Caston SS, Sponseller BA, Dembek KA, et al. Evaluation of locally injected myco-bacterium cell wall fraction in horses with sarcoids. J Equine Vet Sci 2020;90: 103102.
41. Lavach JD, Sullins KE, Roberts SM, et al. BCG treatment of periocular sarcoid. Equine Vet J 1985;17:445–8.
42. Vanselow BA, Abetz I, Jackson AR. BCG emulsion immunotherapy of equine sarcoid. Equine Vet J 1988;20:444–7.
43. Owen RA, Jagger DW. Clinical observations on the use of BCG cell wall fraction for treatment of periocular and other equine sarcoids. Vet Rec 1987;120:548–52.
44. Goodrich L, Gerber H, Marti E, et al. Equine sarcoids. Vet Clin N Am Equine Pract 1998;14:607–23.
45. Hollis AR, Berlato D. Initial experience with High Dose Rate Brachytherapy of periorbital sarcoids in the horse. Equine Vet Educ 2018;30:444–9.
46. Hollis AR. Strontium-90 plesiotherapy in the horse. Equine Vet Educ 2017; 32:7–11.
47. Henson FMD, Dobson JM. Use of radiation therapy in the treatment of equine neoplasia. Equine Vet Educ 2004;16:315–8.
48. Bradley WM, Schlipp D, Khatibzadeh SM. Electronic brachytherapy used for the successful treatment of three different types of equine tumours. Equine Vet Educ 2017;29:293–8.
49. Espy BMK. How to treat equine sarcoids by autologous implantation. Proceed-ings, 54th Annual American Association of Equine Practitioners Convention 2008;68–73.
50. Kinnunen RE, Tallberg T, Stenback H, et al. Equine sarcoid tumour treated by autogenous tumour vaccine. Anticancer Res 1999;19:3367–74.
51. Rothacker CC, Boyle AG, Levine DG. Autologous vaccination for the treatment of equine sarcoids: 18 cases (2009-2014). Can Vet J 2015;56:709–14.
52. Kottenbelt DC, Patterson-Kane JC, Snalune KL. Principles of oncological therapy clinical equine oncology. London: Elsevier; 2015. p. 192–3.
53. Christen-Clottu O, Klocke P, Burger D, et al. Treatment of clinically diagnosed equine sarcoid with a mistletoe extract (Viscum album austriacus). J Vet Intern Med 2010;24:1483–9.
54. Theon AP, Pusterla N, Magdesian KG, et al. A pilot phase II study of the efficacy and biosafety of doxorubicin chemotherapy in tumor-bearing equidae. J Vet Intern Med 2013;27:1581–8.
55. Hollis AR. Managing periocular sarcoids. UK-Vet Equine 2018;2:145–52.
56. Offer KS, Dixon CE, Sutton DGM. Treatment of equine sarcoids: a systematic re-view. Equine Vet J 2023;56(1):12–25.

Squamous Cell Carcinomas in Horses

An Update of the Aetiopathogenesis and Treatment Options

Anna R. Hollis, BVetMed, MSc (Clin Onc), SFHEA, FRCVS

KEYWORDS

- Equine tumor • Squamous cell carcinoma • Metastasis

KEY POINTS

- Squamous cell carcinoma is a multifactorial disease, with ultraviolet exposure, genetic aberrations, and viral infections all implicated in various forms of the disease.
- Metastasis is common, even at the first presentation of the disease, and a 'staging' workup should always be performed at the time of diagnosis.
- Wide surgical excision is the treatment of choice, but recurrences are common despite 'clean' margins of excision.
- Adjunctive treatments such as radiotherapy and chemotherapy may improve the prognosis.

SQUAMOUS CELL CARCINOMA

Squamous cell carcinomas (SCC) are the second most common equine tumor.[1–7] Although it is frequently associated with depigmented skin, it can be found in any skin type and color, and in non-dermatologic locations. The average age at diagnosis varies from 9.9 to 19 years, and the incidence increases with age.[8–11] Metastasis is common, with 6% to 18.6% having metastasis at the first presentation.[9,12–15] Ruling out metastasis via a 'staging workup' should therefore be performed in all cases of equine SCC. Whilst the presence of metastasis does not rule out the possibility of treatment, the prognosis will be worse than in cases where metastasis has not occurred. Anecdotally, metastasis to local lymph nodes is not uncommon. Where these are accessible, the author performs fine needle aspirate of local lymph nodes, with the usual caveats associated with the limited diagnostic accuracy of this

Department of Veterinary Medicine, University of Cambridge, Madingley Road, Cambridge CB3 0ES, UK
E-mail address: arh207@cam.ac.uk

Vet Clin Equine 40 (2024) 421–430
https://doi.org/10.1016/j.cveq.2024.07.007
0749-0739/24/© 2024 Elsevier Inc. All rights reserved, including for text and data mining, AI training, and similar technologies.
vetequine.theclinics.com

approach, to rule in metastasis, counseling owners that you cannot rule out metastasis using this approach.

Chronic exposure to ultraviolet (UV) light is implicated as a risk factor for equine SCC. However, given the diversity of affected anatomic locations, there is more to the disease than chronic UV light exposure. Equine penile SCC is relatively common, representing between 50% and 80% of all external genital neoplasms.[16] Proposed causes include smegma accumulation, chronic irritation, and balanoposthitis.[17] SCC is also the most common neoplasm of the equine stomach.[8] There are also genetic mutations and viral involvement in some forms of SCC in horses. Our understanding of the aetiopathogenesis of SCC continues to evolve.

Ultraviolet Light and Squamous Cell Carcinoma

UV light exposure is a well-documented risk factor for the development of equine SCC, making it easy to explain the predisposition of certain anatomic areas with areas of sun-exposed skin with no pigment. The *TP53* gene leads to the production of tumor protein p53 (*TP53*), which acts as a tumor suppressor, regulating the cell cycle and preventing genome mutation. *TP53* mutations lead primarily to a loss-of-function of p53 protein. This removes intrinsic cellular tumor suppression mechanisms (such as senescence and apoptosis), increasing the risk of cancer.[18] It also reprogrammes cellular metabolism, leading to sustained, continuous tumor cell growth and proliferation.[18,19] Mutations of the p53 tumor suppressor gene can be caused by solar radiation, and have been identified in equine ocular SCC, supporting the role of UV light exposure in these lesions.[20] However, p53 mutations are the most frequently altered gene mutations in human tumors,[18] suggesting that there are other factors affecting the development of this mutation in addition to UV exposure.

Equine Papillomavirus, Inflammation, and Squamous Cell Carcinoma

Chronic inflammation is a well-known risk factor for cancer development and is a feasible mechanism for tumor development in many SCCs in the horse. Equine SCCs have been shown to be associated with an abundant inflammatory infiltrate,[21] supporting the hypothesis that inflammation may be an important part of the etiopathogenesis. The link between human SCC and human papillomavirus (HPV) is well-documented,[22] and there is a similar link between equine SCC and equine papillomavirus-2 (EPV-2).[16,23] SCCs positive for EPV-2 have been found in the genitalia,[24] gastric,[8] and head including the oropharynx.[24,25] The detection rate varies, and not all equine SCC are EPV-2 driven lesions.

The mechanism of papillomavirus-associated carcinogenesis is complex and multi-factorial. In humans, infection with the oncogenic HPV virus leads to dysplastic changes in the cervix and within head and neck tumors.[22,26] However, HPV-associated premalignant changes are more clearly identified in the cervix compared to head and neck tumors, where the role of HPV is less well-understood.[22] HPV onco-genes E6 and E7 drive carcinogenesis by interfering with host cell cycle regulation and apoptosis and are upregulated within HPV-associated tumors.[27] Genetic instability and unregulated cell growth result from these changes, which are fundamental driving forces for the development of neoplasia.[27] EPV-2 E6 upregulation has also been found in equine genital and head SCC,[23] so a similar mechanism may be present in equine lesions.

Genetics and Squamous Cell Carcinoma

Limbal SCC lesions were diagnosed with unusual frequency and at a younger age in Haflingers in the United States of America than would typically be expected.[28]

Analysis showed that affected horses had a shared ancestor, and a missense mutation in damage-specific DNA binding protein 2 (DDB2) was found, demonstrating a genetic risk factor in these animals,[29] and the same risk factor for SCC of the nictitating membrane was also identified.[30] A similar genetic predisposition to limbal SCC has been described in a Rocky Mountain Horse and in Belgian breeds.[31–33] This mutation has not been documented in Arabians or Percherons, and although the risk allele was detected in Appaloosas, a significant association with the development of genital SCC was not found.[31] DDB2 co-operates with other proteins to repair UV-induced DNA damage,[34] so it is logical that a mutation in this protein would not predispose to lesions on the genitalia where UV exposure is less likely. It is possible that Appaloosas with the risk allele might be predisposed to SCC in light-exposed areas, but this has not yet been documented. However, DDB2 affects nucleotide excision repair, apoptosis, and senescence, so mutations in this protein are expected to generally increase the risk of tumor development in addition to its involvement with UV-induced damage repair, and low expression of DDB2 is associated with worse prognoses and higher rates of metastases in colon cancer.[34] Interestingly, DDB2 also affects the sensitivity of cancer cells to radiotherapy and chemotherapy,[34] so knowing that horses have this mutation might also affect treatment choices.

Cyclooxygenase Expression in Equine Squamous Cell Carcinoma

Cyclooxygenase-1 and 2 (COX-1 and COX-2) are frequently upregulated in equine SCCs.[35] Active COX enzymes lead to significant effects on tumorigenesis, including increased angiogenesis and increased metastatic potential.[36] COX-2 expression is well-documented in human tumors, including SCC, and over-expression is associated with a worse response to chemotherapy and radiotherapy, and a worse overall prognosis.[37–40] Components of the COX-prostaglandin pathway are also believed to be important components in tumor initiation.[39] The role of COX-2 over-expression in equine SCC is not yet understood. Improving our understanding of its importance in the initiation and maintenance/progression of equine SCC may give potential therapeutic targets, as well as prognostic information.

Grading of Squamous Cell Carcinoma and Its Clinical Significance

Various grading systems have been used for human SCC,[41] and equine mucocutaneous SCC have been graded in a similar fashion,[10,13,42] with the histologic grading of equine SCC being based on a human grading system.[41] Well-differentiated tumors, G1, have minimal basal/parabasal atypica. Poorly differentiated tumors, G3, have minimal or no architectural similarity with normal tissue. Moderately differentiated tumors, G2, are those not fitting with the criteria described for G1 or G3. SCCs can also be heterogenous, with varying differentiation within the same tumor. Despite this complexity, when applied to equine penile and preputial SCC, the grading appeared to be useful. Metastasis was present with 44% of G3 tumors, compared to 25% of G2, and 3% of G1 lesions, and the histologic grade was associated with the prognosis.[13] Outcomes worsened with increasing grade; 50% of G1 tumors, 75% of G2 tumors, and 80% of G3 tumors had an unsuccessful outcome (recurrence of the lesion, no treatment, or euthanasia). Of those treated, G3 tumors were associated with unfavourable treatment outcomes in 66.7% of cases, compared to 42.9% of G2 and 30.8% of G1 tumors.[13] Metastasis to the regional lymph nodes was associated with recurrence of penile and preputial SCC; 25% of horses with regional lymph node metastasis had recurrence despite treatment.[13]

Overview of Treatment for Equine Squamous Cell Carcinoma

Surgical excision with wide margins is the treatment of choice for all SCC. However, recurrence rates are high, especially with ocular and periocular SCC. There is a 23% to 33% recurrence rate of ocular SCC following surgical excision with clean margins even in humans.[43] Equine data suggest a 30.4% recurrence rate for ocular and periocular lesions, and 11% to 30% recurrence rates for penile and preputial SCC,[13–15,44–46] despite clean margins.

Radiotherapy

Radiotherapy is a useful adjunctive or primary treatment for SCC. Radiotherapy is used as adjunctive therapy in human patients with high-risk histologic features to reduce the risk of recurrence and metastases, and as a sole treatment for human patients who are not suitable for surgery.[47] Radiotherapy is also tissue-preserving and may offer a better cosmetic and functional outcome compared to surgery.[48] Radiotherapy may be suitable for the treatment of equine SCC, with the form chosen dependent on the location and size of the lesion, and the availability of the modality.

There are data to support the use of radiotherapy in equine SCC. Strontium plesiotherapy is a useful adjunctive therapy for equine SCC, especially periocular SCC, where it improved success rates to between 83% and 100%.[49–51] The author has also used this technique to successfully treat a SCC on the lower limb of a horse, which had not responded to surgical excision and topical chemotherapy protocols (**Figs. 1** and **2**). To this author's knowledge, there are no published data relating to the use of high dose rate brachytherapy, electronic brachytherapy, or electrons/photons delivered

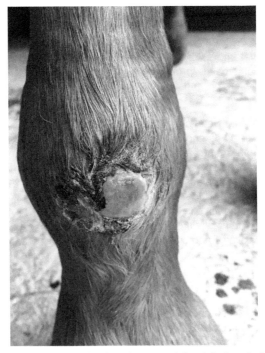

Fig. 1. Confirmed sarcoid lesion on the dorsal aspect of the right fore fetlock, which had not responded to a variety of treatments.

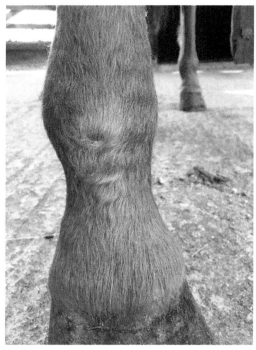

Fig. 2. The same horse as **Fig. 1** and 6 months after strontium plesiotherapy treatment of the lesion. No recurrence has been reported, and the horse is now 7 years post-treatment.

via teletherapy for this tumor type in equine patients. Anecdotal reports support high dose rate brachytherapy and teletherapy in the treatment of equine SCC where these techniques are available.

Chemotherapy

5-fluorouracil (5-FU) has been described for the treatment of SCC of the external genitalia with surgical resection and as a sole treatment,[52] and as a sole treatment to treat other superficial SCCs.[53] Intralesional 5-FU has been used in the treatment of eyelid SCC in 5 horses, but complete resolution was not achieved,[54] so it does not appear to be especially useful in this context.

Cisplatin beads have been used successfully in the management of SCC in a variety of locations.[55] There is also a report of intralesional tigilanol tiglate being successfully used in the management of a single SCC in a horse.[56]

Topical mitomycin C is commonly used for human corneal and conjunctival SCC treatment,[57–63] and in horses success rates of 75% to 90% are reported when used as a sole therapy or in conjunction with surgical excision.[64–66] Various protocols exist in the human literature and can be directly applied to equine treatment, with perhaps the most practical being administering 0.2 mL of 0.04% solution q6h for 7 days on, 7 days off, for up to 4 rounds of treatment. As this is chemotherapy, with associated health and safety implications, this should be administered via a subpalpebral lavage system and in a hospital environment. In humans, pain, swelling, and corneal and scleral melting ulcers have been reported, and these occur more commonly than with other topical treatments such as 5-FU so mitomycin C tends to be reserved for difficult cases that have not responded to other treatment modalities.[62] These have not been reported in the equine literature, and anecdotally, the treatment appears to be well-tolerated in horses.

Topical 5-FU is also commonly used for human ocular SCC,[62] and although it is anecdotally in frequent clinical use in equine cases, there are few reports to support (or refute) its use.[67] In humans there is a complete resolution rate of up to 96% with topical 5-FU when administered q6h for 7 days, followed by 3 weeks of no treatment, with a mean of 4 cycles of treatment administered.[68] Topical 5-FU may lead to side-effects including pain, swelling, and has rarely been associated with stromal melting.[62] Anecdotally, the protocol used in human medicine appears to be effective and practical for use in the horse, although the same precautions as for mitomycin C should be taken – namely, administration via a subpalpebral lavage catheter in a hospital environment.

Other Treatment Modalities

There are weak data to support the use of piroxicam as an adjunctive treatment for equine SCC.[69] In dogs, a small study suggested that piroxicam was as beneficial as cytotoxic therapy,[70] and it has been used in a single equine SCC.[71] Piroxicam is relatively COX-2 specific, and, as already discussed, equine SCC frequently overexpress COX-2, so it is feasible that piroxicam may be of benefit. Firocoxib is another COX-2 specific non-steroidal anti-inflammatory drug with a specific equine license, making it readily available. Firocoxib would therefore be a potentially useful addition to the treatment protocol of equine SCC. If the tumors were routinely analyzed for the expression of COX-2, the treatment could be tailored to those lesions with over-expression and clinical trials could investigate its potential utility for this application.

Other reported therapies for SCC include photodynamic therapy,[72] cryotherapy,[73,74] and radiofrequency hyperthermia[75]; these are mostly used in combination with surgical excision and the very small numbers of cases makes it difficult to interpret results.

SUMMARY

In summary, SCC remains a common tumor type and may be driven by a variety of internal or external factors. Regardless of the etiology, a full staging workup should be performed at the time of diagnosis, as the presence of metastasis may significantly influence the decision-making process for treatment and will undoubtably affect the prognosis.

CLINICS CARE POINTS

- Squamous cell carcinomas are best treated via wide surgical excision wherever possible.
- Recurrence rates are relatively high even following apparently successful excision, so adjunctive treatments are frequently employed to improve the long-term prognosis.
- These are most commonly radiotherapy, where this is available, and topical chemotherapy such as 5-fluorouracil.

DISCLOSURE

The author has no affiliations other than I work for the University of Cambridge.

REFERENCES

1. Valentine BA. Survey of equine cutaneous neoplasia in the Pacific Northwest. J Vet Diagn Invest 2006;18:123–6.
2. Theon AP, Wilson WD, Magdesian KG, et al. Long-term outcome associated with intratumoral chemotherapy with cisplatin for cutaneous tumors in equidae: 573 cases (1995-2004). J Am Vet Med Assoc 2007;230:1506–13.
3. Sundberg JP, Burnstein T, Page EH, et al. Neoplasms of Equidae. J Am Vet Med Assoc 1977;170:150–2.
4. Knowles EJ, Tremaine WH, Pearson GR, et al. A database survey of equine tumours in the United Kingdom. Equine Vet J 2016;48:280–4.
5. Pascoe RR, Summers PM. Clinical survey of tumours and tumour-like lesions in horses in south east Queensland. Equine Vet J 1981;13:235–9.
6. Bastianello SS. A survey on neoplasia in domestic species over a 40-year period from 1935 to 1974 in the Republic of South Africa. IV. Tumours occurring in Equidae. Onderstepoort J Vet Res 1983;50:91–6.
7. Schaffer PA, Wobeser B, Martin LE, et al. Cutaneous neoplastic lesions of equids in the central United States and Canada: 3,351 biopsy specimens from 3,272 equids (2000-2010). J Am Vet Med Assoc 2013;242:99–104.
8. Alloway E, Linder K, May S, et al. A subset of equine gastric squamous cell carcinomas is associated with equus caballus papillomavirus-2 infection. Vet Pathol 2020;57:427–31.
9. King TC, Priehs DR, Gum GG, et al. Therapeutic management of ocular squamous cell carcinoma in the horse: 43 cases (1979-1989). Equine Vet J 1991; 23:449–52.
10. van den Top JG, de Heer N, Klein WR, et al. Penile and preputial squamous cell carcinoma in the horse: a retrospective study of treatment of 77 affected horses. Equine Vet J 2008;40:533–7.
11. Strafuss AC. Squamous cell carcinoma in horses. J Am Vet Med Assoc 1976; 168:61–2.
12. Schwink K. Factors influencing morbidity and outcome of equine ocular squamous cell carcinoma. Equine Vet J 1987;19:198–200.
13. van den Top JG, de Heer N, Klein WR, et al. Penile and preputial tumours in the horse: a retrospective study of 114 affected horses. Equine Vet J 2008;40: 528–32.
14. Mair TS, Walmsley JP, Phillips TJ. Surgical treatment of 45 horses affected by squamous cell carcinoma of the penis and prepuce. Equine Vet Educ 2000;32: 406–10.
15. Howarth S, Lucke VM, Pearson H. Squamous cell carcinoma of the equine external genitalia: a review and assessment of penile amputation and urethrostomy as a surgical treatment. Equine Vet J 1991;23:58.
16. Arthurs C, Suarez-Bonnet A, Willis C, et al. Equine penile squamous cell carcinoma: expression of biomarker proteins and EcPV2. Sci Rep 2020;10:7863.
17. Zhu KW, Affolter VK, Gaynor AM, et al. Equine genital squamous cell carcinoma: in situ hybridization identifies a distinct subset containing equus caballus papillomavirus 2. Vet Pathol 2015;52:1067–72.
18. Mantovani F, Collavin L, Del Sal G. Mutant p53 as a guardian of the cancer cell. Cell Death Differ 2019;26:199–212.
19. Vander Heiden MG, DeBerardinis RJ. Understanding the Intersections between Metabolism and Cancer Biology. Cell 2017;168:657–69.

20. Sironi G, Riccaboni P, Mertel L, et al. p53 protein expression in conjunctival squamous cell carcinomas of domestic animals. Vet Ophthalmol 1999;2:227–31.

21. Perez J, Mozos E, Martin MP, et al. Immunohistochemical study of the inflammatory infiltrate associated with equine squamous cell carcinoma. J Comp Pathol 1999;121:385–97.

22. Brennan S, Baird AM, O'Regan E, et al. The role of human papilloma virus in dictating outcomes in head and neck squamous cell carcinoma. Front Mol Biosci 2021;8:677900.

23. Sykora S, Jindra C, Hofer M, et al. Equine papillomavirus type 2: An equine equivalent to human papillomavirus 16? Vet J 2017;225:3–8.

24. Knight CG, Dunowska M, Munday JS, et al. Comparison of the levels of Equus caballus papillomavirus type 2 (EcPV-2) DNA in equine squamous cell carcinomas and non-cancerous tissues using quantitative PCR. Vet Microbiol 2013; 166:257–62.

25. Pratscher B, Hainisch EK, Sykora S, et al. No evidence of bovine papillomavirus type 1 or 2 infection in healthy equids. Equine Vet J 2019;51:612–6.

26. Maglennon GA, Doorbar J. The biology of papillomavirus latency. Open Virol J 2012;6:190–7.

27. Gheit T. Mucosal and cutaneous human papillomavirus infections and cancer biology. Front Oncol 2019;9:355.

28. Lassaline M, Cranford TL, Latimer CA, et al. Limbal squamous cell carcinoma in Haflinger horses. Vet Ophthalmol 2015;18:404–8.

29. Bellone RR, Liu J, Petersen JL, et al. A missense mutation in damage-specific DNA binding protein 2 is a genetic risk factor for limbal squamous cell carcinoma in horses. Int J Cancer 2017;141:342–53.

30. Singer-Berk M, Knickelbein KE, Vig S, et al. Genetic risk for squamous cell carcinoma of the nictitating membrane parallels that of the limbus in Haflinger horses. Anim Genet 2018;49:457–60.

31. Singer-Berk MH, Knickelbein KE, Lounsberry ZT, et al. Additional evidence for DDB2 T338M as a genetic risk factor for ocular squamous cell carcinoma in horses. Int J Genomics 2019;2019:3610965.

32. Knickelbein KE, Lassaline ME, Singer-Berk M, et al. A missense mutation in damage-specific DNA binding protein 2 is a genetic risk factor for ocular squamous cell carcinoma in Belgian horses. Equine Vet J 2020;52:34–40.

33. Knickelbein KE, Lassaline ME, Bellone RR. Limbal squamous cell carcinoma in a Rocky Mountain Horse: Case report and investigation of genetic contribution. Vet Ophthalmol 2019;22:201–5.

34. Bao N, Han J, Zhou H. A protein with broad functions: damage-specific DNA-binding protein 2. Mol Biol Rep 2022;49:12181–92.

35. Elce YA, Orsini JA, Blikslager AT. Expression of cyclooxygenase-1 and -2 in naturally occurring squamous cell carcinomas in horses. Am J Vet Res 2007;68: 76–80.

36. Elce YA. The aetiopathogenesis of squamous cell carcinomas in horses. Where are we? Equine Vet Educ 2009;21:17–8.

37. Peng L, Zhou Y, Wang Y, et al. Prognostic significance of COX-2 immunohistochemical expression in colorectal cancer: a meta-analysis of the literature. PLoS One 2013;8:e58891.

38. Saito S, Ozawa H, Imanishi Y, et al. Cyclooxygenase-2 expression is associated with chemoresistance through cancer stemness property in hypopharyngeal carcinoma. Oncol Lett 2021;22:533.

39. Greenhough A, Smartt HJ, Moore AE, et al. The COX-2/PGE2 pathway: key roles in the hallmarks of cancer and adaptation to the tumour microenvironment. Carcinogenesis 2009;30:377–86.

40. Pannone G, Bufo P, Caiaffa MF, et al. Cyclooxygenase-2 expression in oral squamous cell carcinoma. Int J Immunopathol Pharmacol 2004;17:273–82.

41. Chaux A, Torres J, Pfannl R, et al. Histologic grade in penile squamous cell carcinoma: visual estimation versus digital measurement of proportions of grades, adverse prognosis with any proportion of grade 3 and correlation of a Gleason-like system with nodal metastasis. Am J Surg Pathol 2009;33:1042–8.

42. van den Top JG, Ensink JM, Barneveld A, et al. Penile and preputial squamous cell carcinoma in the horse and proposal of a classification system. Equine Vet Educ 2011;23:636–48.

43. Rajeh A, Barakat F, Khurma S, et al. Characteristics, management, and outcome of squamous carcinoma of the conjunctiva in a single tertiary cancer center in Jordan. Int J Ophthalmol 2018;11:1132–8.

44. Markel MD, Wheat JD, Jones K. Genital neoplasms treated by en bloc resection and penile retroversion in horses: 10 cases (1977-1986). J Am Vet Med Assoc 1988;192:396–400.

45. Doles J, Williams JW, Yarbrough TB. Penile amputation and sheath ablation in the horse. Vet Surg 2001;30:327–31.

46. Dugan SJ, Curtis CR, Roberts SM, et al. Epidemiologic study of ocular/adnexal squamous cell carcinoma in horses. J Am Vet Med Assoc 1991;198:251–6.

47. Muto P, Pastore F. Radiotherapy in the adjuvant and advanced setting of CSCC. Dermatol Pract Concept 2021;11:e2021168S.

48. Veness MJ, Delishaj D, Barnes EA, et al. Current role of radiotherapy in non-melanoma skin cancer. Clin Oncol 2019;31:749–58.

49. Frauenfelder HC, Blevins WE, Page EH. 90Sr for treatment of periocular squamous cell carcinoma in the horse. J Am Vet Med Assoc 1982;180:307–9.

50. Walker MA, Goble D, Geiser D. Two-year non-recurrence rates for equine ocular and periorbital squamous cell carcinoma following radiotherapy. Vet Radiol 1986; 4:146–8.

51. Plummer CE, Smith S, Andrew SE, et al. Combined keratectomy, strontium-90 irradiation and permanent bulbar conjunctival grafts for corneolimbal squamous cell carcinomas in horses (1990-2002): 38 horses. Vet Ophthalmol 2007;10: 37–42.

52. Fortier LA, Mac Harg MA. Topical use of 5-fluorouracil for treatment of squamous cell carcinoma of the external genitalia of horses: 11 cases (1988-1992). J Am Vet Med Assoc 1994;205:1183–5.

53. Paterson S. Treatment of superficial ulcerative squamous cell carcinoma in three horses with topical 5-fluorouracil. Vet Rec 1997;141:626–8.

54. Pucket JD, Gilmour MA. Intralesional 5-fluorouracil (5-FU) for the treatment of eyelid squamous cell carcinoma in 5 horses. Equine Vet Educ 2014;26:331–5.

55. Hewes CA, Sullins KE. Use of cisplatin-containing biodegradable beads for treatment of cutaneous neoplasia in equidae: 59 cases (2000-2004). J Am Vet Med Assoc 2006;229:1617–22.

56. De Ridder T, Ruppin M, Wheeless M, et al. Use of the intratumoural anticancer drug tigilanol tiglate in two horses. Front Vet Sci 2020;7:639.

57. Panda A, Bajaj MS, Balasubramanya R, et al. Topical mitomycin C for conjunctival-corneal squamous cell carcinoma. Am J Ophthalmol 2003;135: 122–3 [author reply 123-124].

58. Prabhasawat P, Tarinvorakup P, Tesavibul N, et al. Topical 0.002% mitomycin C for the treatment of conjunctival-corneal intraepithelial neoplasia and squamous cell carcinoma. Cornea 2005;24:443–8.

59. Gupta A, Muecke J. Treatment of ocular surface squamous neoplasia with Mitomycin C. Br J Ophthalmol 2010;94:555–8.

60. Poothullil AM, Colby KA. Topical medical therapies for ocular surface tumors. Semin Ophthalmol 2006;21:161–9.

61. Yeoh CHY, Lee JJR, Lim BXH, et al. The management of ocular surface squamous neoplasia (OSSN). Int J Mol Sci 2022;24.

62. Patel U, Karp CL, Dubovy SR. Update on the management of ocular surface squamous neoplasia. Curr Ophthalmol Rep 2021;9:7–15.

63. Monroy D, Serrano A, Galor A, et al. Medical treatment for ocular surface squamous neoplasia. Eye (Lond) 2023;37:885–93.

64. Malalana F. Treatment of periocular tumours - what is the evidence? BEVA congress 2015;66.

65. Clode AB, Miller C, McMullen RJ Jr, et al. A retrospective comparison of surgical removal and subsequent CO2 laser ablation versus topical administration of mitomycin C as therapy for equine corneolimbal squamous cell carcinoma. Vet Ophthalmol 2012;15:254–62.

66. Rayner SG, Van Zyl N. The use of mitomycin C as an adjunctive treatment for equine ocular squamous cell carcinoma. Aust Vet J 2006;84:43–6.

67. Offer KS, Marchesi F, Sutton DGM. Topical 5-fluorouracil as an adjunct treatment in equine corneolimbal squamous cell carcinoma. Equine Vet Educ 2022;34: e363–8.

68. Venkateswaran N, Mercado C, Galor A, et al. Comparison of Topical 5-Fluorouracil and Interferon Alfa-2b as Primary Treatment Modalities for Ocular Surface Squamous Neoplasia. Am J Ophthalmol 2019;199:216–22.

69. Moore AS, Beam SL, Rassnick KM, et al. Long-term control of mucocutaneous squamous cell carcinoma and metastases in a horse using piroxicam. Equine Vet J 2003;35:715–8.

70. Schmidt BR, Glickman NW, DeNicola DB, et al. Evaluation of piroxicam for the treatment of oral squamous cell carcinoma in dogs. J Am Vet Med Assoc 2001;218:1783–6.

71. Moore AS, Wood CA, Engler SJ, et al. Radiation therapy for long-term control of odontogenic tumours and epulis in three cats. J Feline Med Surg 2000;2:57–60.

72. Giuliano EA, MacDonald I, McCaw DL, et al. Photodynamic therapy for the treatment of periocular squamous cell carcinoma in horses: a pilot study. Vet Ophthalmol 2008;11(Suppl 1):27–34.

73. Schoster JV. Using combined excision and cryotherapy to treat limbal squamous cell carcinoma. Vet Med 1992;87.

74. Hilbert BJ, Farrell RK, Grant BD. Cryotherapy of periocular squamous cell carcinoma in the horse. J Am Vet Med Assoc 1977;170:1305–8.

75. Grier RL, Brewer WG Jr, Paul SR, et al. Treatment of bovine and equine ocular squamous cell carcinoma by radiofrequency hyperthermia. J Am Vet Med Assoc 1980;177:55–61.

Equine Melanoma Updates

Anna R. Hollis, BVetMed, MSc (Clin Onc), SFHEA, FRCVS

KEYWORDS

- Melanomatosis • Horse • Tumour

KEY POINTS

- Melanomas are more prevalent in older gray horses; at age 15, 80% of gray horses have at least 1 melanoma.
- Around 66% of lesions will eventually metastasize.
- Melanomas may cause problems locally due to abscessation, ulceration, and interference with function of the affected areas of the body.
- Treatment can be limited by size and location; surgical resection is a better treatment.

MELANOMAS

Melanomas are extremely common in older gray horses, with an increasing risk associated with increasing age and 80% of gray horses have at least 1 melanoma by 15 year old.[1] Although melanomas are typically considered to be a gray horse disease, they can occur sporadically in any color of horse. It is often stated that melanomas occurring in non-grey horses are more aggressive, but this remains anecdotal.

Melanomas have a typical black, round, firm appearance and may progress to ulcerate or abscessate. They can be found in any location but are especially common on the underside of the tail, in the perineal and perigenital region, within the parotid salivary glands, on the eyelids, and on the lips. They occasionally occur within the eye and small lesions often termed 'melanosis' are frequently located on the lining of the guttural pouches. Although equine melanomas are typically considered to be benign, 14% to 66% will eventually metastasize.[2,3] A 5 grade clinical classification system has been proposed,[4] and horses are expected to progress by 0.3 grades per year.

Unfortunately for gray horses, the genetic basis for their coloration predisposes them to the development of melanomas. A genetic mutation causes the coloration. This is a single, 4.6 kB duplication in intron 6 of the *syntaxin-17 (STX17)* gene, causing a melanocyte-specific enhancer upregulated by duplication.[4,5] The duplication of *STX17* boosts expression of *STX17* and its neighboring gene, *NR4A3*, both of which

Department of Veterinary Medicine, University of Cambridge, Madingley Road, Cambridge CB3 0ES, UK
E-mail address: arh207@cam.ac.uk

Vet Clin Equine 40 (2024) 431–439
https://doi.org/10.1016/j.cveq.2024.07.008
0749-0739/24/
vetequine.theclinics.com

enhance proliferation of melanocytes.[5] This leads to premature exhaustion of the stem cell supply that normally progressively depletes during each round of hair growth and shedding, causing progressive pileous depigmentation and graying of hair follicles and the typical color, which becomes more 'white' with increasing age.[5] However, this same overproliferation of melanocytes may predispose the animal to neoplastic transformation and the development of melanomas. The gray-inducing STX17 mutation, STX17^G, is found within equine melanomas, with copy number expansions of STX17^G found in 5 of 8 melanomas, and a tendency toward increasing copy numbers in more aggressive tumors.[6]

The grey-inducing STX17^G (G) is autosomal dominant and is epistatic for coat color. This means that horses of any base color with STX17^G at 1 or both alleles (G/g or G/G) will become gray.[4] Interestingly, STX17^G also influences vitiligo and speckling of the gray coat. Horses with 2 copies of the mutation (G/G) will gray out more quickly and completely, have more vitiligo of hairless skin, less speckling of the gray coat, and greater prevalence and severity of melanomas.[7] One cohort of 1119 gray Lipizzaner horses found that an additional copy of STX17^G was associated with an increase in melanoma grading by 0.85/5.[4]

Other genes also affect the risk of melanoma development. The agouti signaling protein reduces MC1R activation through interference with the binding of alpha-melanocyte-stimulating hormone (α-MSH). Agouti signaling protein is encoded by ASIP^A, with loss-of-function recessive alleles being ASIP^a, and horses with mutant ASIP do not have this normal inhibition of α-MSH. Melanocortin-1 receptor is encoded by MC1R^E with the dominant allele enabling synthesis of the black hair pigment eumelanin, and the loss-of-function recessive alleles being MC1R^e, which cause the chestnut coat color and which may also hypothetically reduce the risk of melanoma.[8] As both the STX17^G mutation and signaling through MC1R promote melanocyte proliferation, the ASIP^a mutation-driven unrestricted MCR1 activation may increase the risk of melanoma. This has been seen in Lipizzaners, where each copy of the ASIP^a mutation increased the melanoma grade by 0.19/5 (so homozygotes had a grade 0.38/5 higher than those without this mutation).[4] Theoretically, based on these color genetics, the relative risk for the development of melanoma based on pre-graying coat color is black >bay>chestnut.[8]

There may also be a breed-dependent effect on melanoma prevalence. The prevalence in horses older than 15 years has been reported to be 68% in Carmargue, 75% in Lipizzaners, and 100% in Pura Raza Espanola (PRE), compared to 52% of gray Quarter Horses of the same age.[2,8–11] The gray coat color is predominant or breed-defining in Lipizzaners, PRE, and Carmague, and the MC1R chestnut allele is absent or extremely low frequency in these breeds.[5] In contrast, there is a high frequency of the chestnut allele in gray Quarter Horses, and there is apparently reduced melanoma prevalence. This could be because of infrequent homozygosity of STX17, a mitigating effect of the common MC1R mutation on the ASIP potentiation of melanoma, other genes in the MC1R signaling pathway, or other differences in genetics as yet undefined.[8]

Progression of Melanomas

Most melanomas start as a small raised black cutaneous nodule or plaque in an area of hairless skin.[7] Progression is variable, but generally involves a combination of spread of existing tumors (local, lymphatic, or vascular spread), and/or emergence of new melanomas.[7] As tumors grow and coalesce they may affect the structure and function of surrounding areas, for example, perianal and perineal tumors may cause dyschezia and rectal impactions. Rapidly growing tumors may outgrow their blood supply, leading to the development of (usually central) necrosis and sterile abscessation, which typically have a black, tarry liquid content. Whilst systemic malignancy tends to occur late in the disease process, locoregional malignancy is more likely to be problematic. The grading system proposed by Curik and colleagues[4] is a useful tool to assist with the staging of the disease and to explain the likely progression to owners, with horses frequently progressing by 1 grade approximately every 3 years (**Table 1**). However, this does appear to be breed-dependent, with breeds selected for gray coat color, such as the Lipizzaner, progressing more rapidly than breeds not usually selected for gray coat color, such as the Quarter Horse.[4,5]

Treatment of Melanomas

Surgical excision, where possible, is the mainstay of melanoma treatment.[7] This is expected to be locally curative with minimal complications, even where lesions are large and/or coalescing.[12] When surgical margins were clear, tumor regrowth appeared to be unlikely – in a case series of 38 melanomas ranging from 4 cm to 20 cm removed surgically; none regrew at the surgical site, with follow-up of up to 163 mo.[12] Given the mechanism of melanoma development, it is not surprising that surgical excision did not appear to have any impact on the continued growth of remaining masses.[12] Despite this, the successful removal of lesions up to 20 cm in diameter with few or no complications makes this an attractive option in the majority of cases.[12] In a case series, 10 large tumors had adjunctive treatment using cisplatin beads, and none recurred in the 12 months after surgery.[12]

Intralesional Treatments for Melanomas

Melanoma cells appear to be relatively resistant to systemic cytotoxic chemotherapy, but intralesional treatment with platinum-based chemotherapy agents (cisplatin and carboplatin) may be effective.[13] Cisplatin and carboplatin beads may be surgically implanted alongside or within nodules, which may lead to regression.[14] Larger lesions (in excess of 2 cm diameter) are usually removed or debulked surgically prior to adjunctive treatments, where cisplatin or carboplatin emulsion or biodegradable beads may be placed into the wound margins.[12,14] Because of the health and safety implications of platinum based chemotherapy, it is this author's preference to use surgical excision alone as there is currently insufficient data to suggest there is a benefit associated with the addition of chemotherapy. Some clinicians are using other intralesional agents, such as mitomycin C and tigilanol tiglate, and these agents may also

Table 1	
Proposed grading system for classification of melanoma	
Grade of Disease	**Description**
0	No melanomas present
1	Early stage, plaque type, single <0.5 cm nodule in a typical location
2	Several 0.5 cm nodules or a single <2 cm nodule in typical locations
3	One or several nodules <5 cm, intra- or subcutaneous, typical locations or on lips
4	Extensive confluent subcutaneous melanomas with necrosis and/or ulceration, or metastasis
5	Exophytic tumor growth with wet surfaces and ulceration, metastasis with associated clinical signs (cachexia, fever, etc)

Adapted from Curik et al (2013).[4]

be considered in more difficult cases, although there are minimal data supporting (or refuting) their utility in equine melanomas at this time. Intralesional mitomycin C has been described as part of treatment for a corneal melanoma in one horse, but it is difficult to draw any definitive conclusion on its utility as it was part of multimodal therapy, and there was only very short-term follow-up.[15]

Amblyomin-X is a recombinant protein from the tick *Amblyomma sculptum*, which triggers apoptosis by activating an intrinsic pathway within tumor cells.[16] Amblyomin-X has been investigated for use in equine melanomas, although the focus of the study was as a model for human melanomas, rather than as a treatment for horses,[16] making it harder to interpret. This study had both an in vivo and an ex vivo component. In the in vivo part, 4 horses with 9 tumors per case were included. Three tumors were treated with intralesional amblyomin-X, 3 were injected with placebo, and 3 were not treated on each horse (12 treated with the drug, 12 with placebo, and 12 not treated in total). The injection was given at 1 mg/kg of tumor mass every 3 days for 28 days, and there were 5 months of follow-up. All treated lesions reduced in size, and some regressed completely. In the ex vivo part of the study, 12 further tumors were injected at the same dose rate and then excised 6 to 12 hours later (6 tumors at 6 h, and 6 tumors at 12 h). There was a modulated tumor microenvironment following treatment in all excised tumors.[16] The study was not aiming to provide the data on the treatment of equine melanomas for the benefit of the horse, but instead as a potential human treatment. However, this is an interesting treatment which shows promise.

Electrochemotherapy for Melanomas

Electrochemotherapy uses electrical pulses applied across tumors to open transient pores in cell membranes, propelling drug molecules into the cytosol. This leads to increased cytotoxicity of substances, with the toxicity of bleomycin being increased up to 8000-fold, and that of cisplatin up to 80-fold.[7] The procedure is usually performed under general anesthetic, and electrochemotherapy is performed immediately after the lesion is saturated with cisplatin, carboplatin, or bleomycin. There are limited literatures suggesting that this approach may be useful for melanomas.[17–19] One of these cases only achieved local control of the disease for 5 mo, and the horse was euthanased 7 mo after the first electrochemotherapy treatment due to abdominal metastases.[18] Another case was lost to follow-up at 12 months when partial remission had been achieved.[17] In a small case series, 8 melanomas (on 8 horses) were treated with electrochemotherapy alone, of which only 2 lesions achieved a complete response at 24 and 36 mo, respectively. Of the other 6 cases, 1 had stable disease at 7 mo, and 5 had a partial response at between 12 to 48 mo post-treatment.[19] In contrast, a single melanoma in the same case series was treated with a combination of surgical excision and electrochemotherapy, and the horse had no evidence of disease at 24 mo.[19] Based on the available data, it is hard to draw definitive conclusions as to the utility of electrochemotherapy in equine melanomas, especially considering the high success rates associated with surgical excision. However, it may be an option for cases that are not amenable to surgical resection.

Hyperthermia for Melanomas

Hyperthermia leads to antitumour effects via multiple pathways, including overexpression of heat shock proteins and shedding of molecules expressing damage-associated molecular patterns, which boost innate and acquired antitumour responses.[20] It may also potentiate the cytotoxicity of chemotherapeutic agents.

Hyperthermia can be achieved with ultrasound, radiofrequency, or microwave energy, and 1 system of microwave energy has been successfully used for the treatment of melanomas in horses.[21] This used 2 rounds of 30 to 60 min of hyperthermia after intralesional cisplatin or carboplatin, which was repeated every 2 weeks. This was used for both debulked tumors and on 2 large lesions that had not undergone surgical debulking, with apparently good results.[21] It is unclear that this was benefit over surgery or intralesional chemotherapy alone.

Radiotherapy for Melanomas

In general, melanomas are relatively radioresistant. The usual caveats of the cost and limited availability of radiotherapy also apply. However, an extensive preputial melanoma has been successfully treated using electronic brachytherapy combined with surgical debulking,[22] so its use could be considered in appropriate cases.

Immunotherapy for Melanomas

Cimetidine inhibits the suppressive action of regulatory T lymphocytes. Cimetidine administered to horses at 1.6 to 7.5 mg/kg/day appeared to lead to regression of melanomas in a small number of horses, but subsequent case series were unable to confirm these findings.[23–26] When cimetidine is used in human oncology, doses are far higher, and if the same magnitude of increase were applied to the equine dose, 48 to 72 mg/kg/d would need to be administered.[27] It is possible that consistently good results would be seen if horses were treated with these doses; however, the cost would be prohibitive.

Interleukins (IL) 12 and 18 are cytokines that stimulate innate and acquired immune responses and have been described. Equine melanomas were injected 1 to 6 times with equine or human IL-12, equine IL-18, or a combination of equine IL-12 and equine IL-18, and in all cases there was a reduction in the lesion size, although resolution was not achieved.[28–30] Shrinkage was observed in noninjected lesions in horses treated with both intralesional and intramuscular IL-12 in combination with IL18.[30] Although these results are interesting, the approach has not found widespread clinical use, probably because of limited availability and high cost.

Autologous vaccines may be useful. In a case series of 12 horses, 11 horses were found to have regression of their melanomas following administration of a whole-cell autogenous vaccination, although data regarding the duration of follow-up and the extent of regression were not reported.[31]

Other vaccination strategies have been explored for melanomas. Melanocytes express surface membrane disialoganglioside GD2 and GD3, which are potential vaccination targets, with anti-GD2 and anti-GD3 monoclonal antibodies enhancing cytotoxicity against canine melanoma cell lines.[32] Dogs vaccinated with an anti-GD3 vaccine generate antibody and cell-mediated immune responses,[33] but these vaccines are not in routine clinical use. A small number of horses vaccinated with the same vaccine showed no significant change in the size of 55 melanomas in 14 horses over a 1 to 2 year period, but the lack of an untreated control group and widely ranging data make it difficult to interpret these results.[7]

A single horse with 'high grade' melanoma has been injected with 8 doses of a DNA plasmid vaccination containing the Streptococcus pyogenes emm55 gene, which led to shrinking of all tumors, including those not injected, and a demonstrable antimelanoma IgG antibody response.[34] Although these are exciting data, to the author's knowledge, no further reports on this approach have been published.

One vaccine that has made it into routine clinical use in dogs is a DNA vaccine against tyrosinase (the Oncept canine melanoma vaccine). This bacterial plasmid vaccine encodes the human tyrosinase gene, and tyrosinase is expressed at high levels in equine melanomas. In addition, the vaccine is safe in horses, and generates a robust antibody and cell-mediated response against equine tyrosinase.[21] Anecdotally, 'most horses demonstrated tumor shrinkage after vaccination',[21] although that is not this author's experience, nor that of a group who presented some data at the European College Equine Internal Medicine Congress in 2022. This group found that vaccinated horses showed no significant increase in melanoma tumor volumes over a 231 day follow-up period, compared to melanomas in untreated horses, which did increase in size over a 126 day follow-up period, but tumor regression was not found.[35] There are potential confounding factors with this study, and to date it remains unpublished except in abstract form, but it does demonstrate that the vaccination may be useful at preventing worsening of the disease. This is consistent with the present author's experience, where several horses have been treated with the Oncept melanoma vaccine for many years without evidence of any disease progression (Hollis, 2024, unpublished data). Disappointingly, the inclusion of the human tyrosinase gene in a DNA minimal vector in combination with IL-12 and IL-18 found no advantage over a combination of IL-12 and IL-18 alone.[30] In addition, in 4 cases of intraocular melanoma, 2 cases progressed and 2 cases appear to have improved following Oncept vaccination.[36] As this is an immune-based vaccine and the eye is an immune privileged site, it is perhaps surprising that there was any benefit in any case; this may have been possible because of the abnormalities associated with the neoplastic lesions affecting the normal 'immune privilege' of the eye. Regardless, it is difficult to draw any conclusions from the limited data presently available on Oncept in horses. There is clearly the need for a multicentre, international effort to consistently document and follow cases over a long time period, but it is a commercially available and potentially useful treatment.

Betulinic Acid

Betulinic acid is a triterpenoid extracted from white birch bark. It permeates equine skin in vitro, and has anti-cancer activity against equine melanoma cells through anti-proliferative and cytotoxic effects.[37] It may therefore be useful in the treatment of equine melanomas. It is safe and well-tolerated when used topically in healthy horses, with only mild local effects seen.[38] Both betulinic acid and its derivative, NVX-207, have been used topically for the treatment of 207 melanomas in 18 horses, and the betulinic acid treated tumors showed a statistically significant decrease in size over a 91 day treatment period, not observed in placebo treated lesions.[39] The lesions treated with NVX-207 did not show a statistically significant decrease in size.[39] These early results show promise, although the treated lesions were all relatively small. More work is required before this treatment could be recommended clinically, but it may prove to be a useful, practical treatment for accessible lesions.

What Is the Future for Equine Melanoma Treatment?

There is no consensus on the best strategy for treatment of equine melanoma. It is this author's belief that based on the currently available data, easily accessible cutaneous masses should be routinely excised to prevent progression, and that clients should be counseled to expect development of new lesions. The use of the Oncept melanoma vaccine can be considered as an adjunctive strategy, aiming to reduce the rate of progression of the disease. There are currently limited data to support this or any other approaches, and further work is urgently needed to progress our understanding of the disease and its treatments.

CLINICS CARE POINTS

- Based on the current clinical evidence, melanomas should be excised as early as possible to prevent progression. Where surgical excision is not possible, intralesional treatments with mitomycin C or tigilanol tiglate are potential treatment options.

- The Oncept melanoma vaccine is an interesting potential treatment. There are few data either supporting or refuting its use. The author believes that it appears to have a role to stabilise disease, reducing the rate of progression, but that it is not appropriate for the treatment of advanced disease because lesion regression appears to be extremely unlikely following treatment.

DISCLOSURE

The author has no affiliations other than her work for the University of Cambridge.

REFERENCES

1. Valentine BA. Equine melanocytic tumors: a retrospective study of 53 horses (1988 to 1991). J Vet Intern Med 1995;9:291–7.
2. Seltenhammer MH, Heere-Ress E, Brandt S, et al. Comparative histopathology of grey-horse-melanoma and human malignant melanoma. Pigm Cell Res 2004;17: 674–81.
3. MacGillivray KC, Sweeney RW, Del Piero F. Metastatic melanoma in horses. J Vet Intern Med 2002;16:452–6.
4. Curik I, Druml T, Seltenhammer M, et al. Complex inheritance of melanoma and pigmentation of coat and skin in Grey horses. PLoS Genet 2013;9:e1003248.
5. Rosengren Pielberg G, Golovko A, Sundstrom E, et al. A cis-acting regulatory mutation causes premature hair graying and susceptibility to melanoma in the horse. Nat Genet 2008;40:1004–9.
6. Sundstrom E, Imsland F, Mikko S, et al. Copy number expansion of the STX17 duplication in melanoma tissue from Grey horses. BMC Genom 2012;13:365.
7. Mackay RJ. Treatment options for melanoma of grey horses. Vet Clin North Am Eq Pract 2019;35:311–25.
8. Teixeira RB, Rendahl AK, Anderson SM, et al. Coat color genotypes and risk and severity of melanoma in gray quarter horses. J Vet Intern Med 2013;27:1201–8.
9. Fleury C, Berard F, Leblond A, et al. The study of cutaneous melanomas in Camargue-type gray-skinned horses (2): epidemiological survey. Pigm Cell Res 2000;13:47–51.
10. Fleury C, Berard F, Balme B, et al. The study of cutaneous melanomas in Camargue-type gray-skinned horses (1): clinical-pathological characterization. Pigm Cell Res 2000;13:39–46.
11. Rodriguez F, Garcia-Barona V, Pena L, et al. Grey horse melanotic condition: a pigmentary disorder. J Vet Eq Vet Sci 1997;17:677–81.
12. Groom LM, Sullins KE. Surgical excision of large melanocytic tumours in grey horses: 38 cases (2001–2013). Equine Vet Educ 2018;30:438–43.
13. Theon AP. Intralesional and topical chemotherapy and immunotherapy. Vet Clin North Am Eq Pract 1998;14:659–71.
14. Hewes CA, Sullins KE. Use of cisplatin-containing biodegradable beads for treatment of cutaneous neoplasia in equidae: 59 cases (2000-2004). J Am Vet Med Assoc 2006;229:1617–22.

15. Strauss RA, Allbaugh RA, Haynes J, et al. Primary corneal malignant melanoma in a horse. Equine Vet Educ 2019;31:403–9.

16. Lichtenstein F, Iqbal A, de Lima WS, et al. Modulation of stress and immune response by Amblyomin-X results in tumor cell death in a horse melanoma model. Sci Rep 2020;10:6388.

17. Spugnini EP, D'Alterio GL, Eng ID, et al. Electrochemotherapy for the treatment of multiple melanomas in a horse. J Eq Vet Sci 2011;31:430–3.

18. Scacco L, Bolaffio CB, Romano A, et al. Adjuvant electrochemotherapy increases local control in a recurring equine anal melanoma. J Vet Eq Sci 2013;33:637–9.

19. Spugnini EP, Scacco L, Bolaffio CB, et al. Electrochemotherapy for the treatment of cutaneous solid tumours in equids: a retrospective study. Open Vet J 2021;11: 385–9.

20. Mahmood J, Shukla HD, Soman S, et al. Immunotherapy, Radiotherapy, and Hyperthermia: A Combined Therapeutic Approach in Pancreatic Cancer Treatment. Cancers 2018;10.

21. Phillips JC, Lembcke LM. Equine melanocytic tumours. Vet Clin North Am Eq Pract 2013;29:673–87.

22. Bradley WM, Schlipp D, Khatibzadeh SM. Electronic brachytherapy used for the successful treatment of three different types of equine tumours. Equine Vet Educ 2017;29:293–8.

23. Goetz TE, Ogilvie GK, Keegan KG, et al. Cimetidine for treatment of melanomas in three horses. J Am Vet Med Assoc 1990;196:449–52.

24. Goetz TE, Long MT. Treatment of melanomas in horses. Compend Contin Educ Vet 1993;15:608–10.

25. Hare JE, Staempfli HR. Cimetidine for the treatment of melanomas in horses - efficacy determined by client questionnaire. Equine Pract 1994;16.

26. Laus F, Cerquetella M, Paggi E. Evaluation of cimetidine as a therapy for dermal melanomatosis in grey horse. Refu Vet 2010;65:48–52.

27. Smyth GB, Duran S, Ravis W, et al. Pharmacokinetic studies of cimetidine hydrochloride in adult horses. Equine Vet J 1990;22:48–50.

28. Heinzerling LM, Feige K, Rieder S, et al. Tumor regression induced by intratumoral injection of DNA coding for human interleukin 12 into melanoma metastases in gray horses. J Mol Med (Berl) 2001;78:692–702.

29. Muller J, Feige K, Wunderlin P, et al. Double-blind placebo-controlled study with interleukin-18 and interleukin-12-encoding plasmid DNA shows antitumor effect in metastatic melanoma in gray horses. J Immunother 2011;34:58–64.

30. Mahlmann K, Feige K, Juhls C, et al. Local and systemic effect of transfection-reagent formulated DNA vectors on equine melanoma. BMC Vet Res 2015; 11:132.

31. Phillips J. Melanoma. In: Sprayberry KA, Robinson NE, editors. Current therapy in equine medicine, 7th edition. 2015. St Louis (MO): p. 524–528.

32. Almela RM, Anson A. A Review of Immunotherapeutic Strategies in Canine Malignant Melanoma. Vet Sci 2019;6.

33. Milner RJ, Salute M, Crawford C, et al. The immune response to disialoganglioside GD3 vaccination in normal dogs: a melanoma surface antigen vaccine. Vet Immunol Immunopathol 2006;114:273–84.

34. Brown EL, Vijayakumar KR, Wright CA, et al. Treatment of metastatic equine melanoma with a plasmid DNA vaccine encoding Streptococcus pyogenes EMM55 protein. J Vet Eq Sci 2014;34:704–8.

35. Echelmeyer J, Peckary R, Delarocque J, et al. Effect of vaccination with human tyrosinase DNA in horses with melanoma in comparison to untreated horses. J Vet Intern Med 2021;35:666–83.
36. Halliwell E, Carslake H, Malalana F. Vaccination with human tyrosinase DNA as a therapy for equine intraocular melanoma - 4 cases: 2016-2021. Equine Vet Educ 2023;35:e234–40.
37. Weber LA, Meissner J, Delarocque J, et al. Betulinic acid shows anticancer activity against equine melanoma cells and permeates isolated equine skin in vitro. BMC Vet Res 2020;16:44.
38. Weber LA, Puff C, Kalbitz J, et al. Concentration profiles and safety of topically applied betulinic acid and NVX-207 in eight healthy horses-A randomized, blinded, placebo-controlled, crossover pilot study. J Vet Pharmacol Therapeut 2021;44:47–57.
39. Weber LA, Delarocque J, Feige K, et al. Effects of Topically Applied Betulinic Acid and NVX-207 on Melanocytic Tumors in 18 Horses. Animals (Basel) 2021;11.

Lymphoma & Myeloproliferative Disease

Amanda Samuels, VMD, PhD, Teresa A. Burns, DVM, PhD*

KEYWORDS

- Lymphoma • Leukemia • Myeloproliferative • Bone marrow • Lymph node
- Chemotherapy

KEY POINTS

- Lymphoma is not restricted to geriatric horses; the median age at diagnosis is 10 to 13 years old.
- Mucocutaneous (skin, nasal mucosa, and nasopharyngeal) lymphoma can present as discrete masses or multiple masses, but the presentation may depend upon the specific lymphoma subtype. Biopsy is critical for diagnosis and to rule out non-neoplastic lesions. Treatments include surgical removal and local chemotherapy. Prognosis is generally favorable.
- Alimentary lymphoma often causes chronic clinical signs: diarrhea, weight loss, and intermittent colic. Research in companion animals suggests that alimentary lymphoma may exist on a spectrum with inflammatory bowel disease. Useful diagnostic tests include rectal palpation, transabdominal ultrasound, and rectal/duodenal biopsies. Treatments include systemic immunosuppression (corticosteroids) and/or cytotoxic chemotherapy. Prognosis depends upon the subtype, treatment, and timing of intervention.
- Other anatomic locations of lymphoma (including multicentric, central nervous system, mediastinal, hepatosplenic, and mesenteric) are associated with clinical signs consistent with the organ system(s) involved. Useful diagnostic tests include rectal palpation, transabdominal ultrasound, and biopsy. Treatment includes systemic immunosuppression (corticosteroids) and/or cytotoxic chemotherapy. Prognosis is generally guarded to poor for long-term survival.
- Leukemias are rare in horses; however, the most commonly reported are acute lymphocytic leukemia (ALL), acute myelocytic leukemia (AML), and chronic lymphocytic leukemia (CLL). ALL tends to affect younger horses (2–8 years), and CLL tends to affect older horses (14–20 years). Clinical signs often include persistent/intermittent fever, lethargy, and lymphadenopathy. Useful diagnostic tests include bone marrow biopsy and complete blood count. Treatment is systemic immunosuppression and cytotoxic chemotherapy. Prognosis depends on the tumor subtype and whether treatment is pursued.

Department of Veterinary Clinical Sciences, College of Veterinary Medicine, The Ohio State University, Columbus, OH, USA
* Corresponding author. 601 Vernon L. Tharp Street, Columbus, OH, 43210.
E-mail address: burns.402@osu.edu

Vet Clin Equine 40 (2024) 441–454
https://doi.org/10.1016/j.cveq.2024.07.009   **vetequine.theclinics.com**

LYMPHOMA

Lymphomas arise from the clonal proliferation of B-cells, T-cells, and natural killer cells and are classified on a cellular level based on maturity and lineage. Recent survey studies indicate that lymphoma is the second most common malignant neoplasm in the horse,[1,2] with 14 different subtypes.[3] For the equine practitioner, classifying lymphoma based on anatomic location may help to provide prognostic and therapeutic options to the owner. There are 3 main anatomic characterizations of lymphoma in horses: multicentric, mucocutaneous, and alimentary, with multicentric being the most common.[3–5]

Lymphoma has also been described in the thoracic cavity,[6] nervous system,[7] nasal/oral cavity,[3,8,9] pelvis,[10] bladder,[11] and ocular/orbital region.[3,12] For this review, the discussion is focused on the most common anatomic locations, but it is important to be aware that the clinical signs associated with rare forms of lymphoma reflect the organ system that is primarily affected and thus can be diverse.

Equine lymphoma may be challenging to diagnose due to the potential diversity of presenting signs and inconsistent diagnostic findings. Particularly with alimentary and multicentric lymphoma, horses often present with non-specific signs.[5,12–14] The mean age of horses diagnosed with lymphoma ranges from 5[5] to 16 years.[13] Most reports find that the mean age of horses diagnosed with lymphoma is 10 to 13 years.[2,3,14,15] Most reports do not separate the mean age based on anatomic distribution; therefore, it is possible that certain anatomic variants may be associated with unique mean ages—this warrants further investigation.

The following section contains descriptions of common clinical presentations, highlights useful diagnostic tests, and provides information regarding treatment and prognosis. The goal is to provide equine practitioners with tools to diagnose lymphoma in equine patients and guide horse owners through the process of treatment and end-of-life decisions.

MULTICENTRIC LYMPHOMA

Multicentric lymphoma is the most common form of the disease in horses,[3–5,16] and based on 2 reports, the most common subtypes are T-cell lymphoma[5] and T-cell-rich large B-cell lymphoma (TCRLBCL).[3] To be classified as multicentric, at least 2 organs need to be involved, including lymph nodes. Organs involved can include the liver, spleen, intestine, kidney, lung, and bone marrow, among others.[7,17–19] The mean age of diagnosis and breed predilections are unclear. In one case series, Quarter Horses were more frequently diagnosed compared to other breeds; however, in this same report, Quarter Horses were also the most common breed.[3]

Clinical Presentation and Diagnostic Testing

Clinical presentation mirrors the organs involved and importantly, multiple organ systems can be affected.[7,11,17–21] Based on limited reports, the most common clinical signs include edema, weight loss, lethargy, and anorexia.[3,5]

Diagnostic testing should be guided by clinical signs and often, blood work is low-yield and frequently reflects the degree of systemic disease.[7,11,16,21] In one case series, the most consistent clinicopathologic findings were decreased albuminconcentration and increased globulins concentration[5] but did not separate lymphoma based on anatomic location. Another report specifically analyzing multicentric lymphoma found equal prevalence of horses with low, normal, and high globulins concentrations.[16] The most fruitful diagnostic tests are commonly transcutaneous ultrasound, rectal palpation, and biopsies of any abnormal organ identified on rectal palpation or ultrasound. Histopathology in conjunction with immunohistochemistry (IHC) should be pursued, since prognosis can vary with different subtypes.[4,16]

Treatment and Prognosis

Treatment protocols are likely comparable to those recommended for alimentary lymphoma and importantly, to date, reports in the equine literature have not separated treatment protocols based on anatomic location.[4,5,16] The authors suggest that until additional research clarifies this question, multicentric and alimentary lymphoma will likely be treated with similar chemotherapeutic protocols (**Table 1**). Although individual treatment protocols were not reported in 1 paper, response to treatment was variable: 2 horses had complete remission, 9 had a partial response, and 1 had stable disease.[4]

Based on the literature, multicentric lymphoma carries a worse prognosis than other forms, with the median survival time being 6 days in one report.[16] However, it is important to note that the range was 1 to 4001 days, which could reflect different organ involvement, whether or not treatment was pursued, and the stage of disease when identified. This information was not available. Another report found a median survival time of 7 months when horses were treated with cytotoxic chemotherapy.[4]

Mucocutaneous lymphoma

Cutaneous neoplasia is common in equine species[22,23]; however, lymphoma is less common than sarcoid, squamous cell carcinoma, and melanoma. Based on 3 survey studies characterizing cutaneous neoplasms, the frequency of cutaneous lymphoma ranges from 1.7% to 4.0%.[22–24] However, the 3 studies originate from the Pacific and Central United States and Canada, and it is unknown whether the prevalence varies by geographic region.

The most common subtype of mucocutaneous lymphoma is TCRLBCL,[16,25] followed by cutaneous T-cell lymphoma (CTCL).[25] A breed predilection might exist; in a survey of cutaneous lymphomas, 96% of the affected Quarter Horses had TCRLBCL. In Thoroughbreds, TCRLBCL was the most common subtype, but the frequency of CTCL was higher compared to other breeds.[25] Studies on equine lymphoma rarely separate age and anatomic distribution. However, based on a few reports, the average age of horses diagnosed with mucocutaneous lymphoma ranges from 6 to 18 years.[26,27]

Clinical Presentation

Nodules are typically firm, well-circumscribed, and non-painful.[28] The nodules can present as either multiple masses in varying locations (including the neck, shoulder, limbs, and scrotum) or as solitary masses that can be found throughout the body (including nictitans).[12,25,27,29] Typically, horses do not show systemic abnormalities, unless the tumor is found in locations associated with specific clinical signs.[27,30,31]

The most common presentation of TCRLBCL is multiple subcutaneous nodules that can range in size from 2 cm to greater than 4 cm.[3,25] TCRLBCL is often found on the head and neck, and in a survey study, all lesions on horses bearing multiple subcutaneous nodules were identified as TCRLBCL.[25] Some reports describe TCRLBCL to have a waxing and waning course[32] and have observed progesterone receptors expressed in 64% of TCRLBCL.[33] The most common presentation of CTCL is a single solitary mass.[25]

Diagnostic Testing

Biopsy is the diagnostic test of choice for nodular lesions and can include excision, punch, or wedge biopsy. Subsequent processing for IHC is important to determine

Table 1
Drugs used in the treatment of hematopoietic malignancy in horses[4,30,74-76]

Drug	Dose	Route	Frequency	Potential Toxicity
Actinomycin-D	0.5–0.75 mg/m²[a]	IV (strictly)	Every 3 wk	BMS; tissue necrosis with extravasation
L-Asparaginase	10,000–40,000 IU/m²	IM or SC	Every 2–3 wk	Hypersensitivity
Azathioprine	3 mg/kg	PO	Every 24 h	Immunosuppression
Chlorambucil	20–30 mg/m²	PO	Every 2 wk	BMS
Cyclophosphamide	200–800 mg/m²	IV	Every 1–2 wk	BMS; hemorrhagic cystitis
Cytosine arabinoside	200–300 mg/m²	SC, IM, IV	Every 1–2 wk	
Dexamethasone	0.05–0.2 mg/kg	PO, IM, IV	Every 24 h	Laminitis, PU/PD, immunosuppression
Diphenhydramine	0.5–1.0 mg/kg	IV or IM	Premedication before drugs associated with hypersensitivity	Excitation; seizure; muscle tremor (less likely with IM route)
Doxorubicin	30–65 mg/m² (cumulative dose restricted to 500 mg/m² in humans)	IV (strictly)	Every 3 wk	Hypersensitivity; nephrotoxicity; cardiotoxicity; tissue necrosis with extravasation
Flunixin meglumine	1.1 mg/kg	IV or PO	Premedication before drugs associated with hypersensitivity; every 12–24 h	GI ulceration; nephrotoxicity
Lomustine (CCNU)	65 mg/m²	IG	Every 4 wk	BMS
Prednisolone	1–2 mg/kg	PO or IV	Every 24–48 h	Laminitis, PU/PD, immunosuppression
Vincristine	0.5–0.7 mg/m²	IV	Weekly	BMS

Abbreviations: BMS, bone marrow suppression; IG, intragastrically via nasogastric tube; IM, intramuscularly; IU, international units; IV, intravenously; PO, per os; PU/PD, polyuria/polydipsia; SC, subcutaneously.
[a] Body surface area (m²) = weight (g²ᐟ³) × 10.5.

the origin (B-cell or T-cell), as the prognosis can differ.[5,25,26] The only bloodwork finding that has been associated with cutaneous lymphoma is globulins concentration, where a report found that 37% of horses had low or normal globulins; none of the horses had high globulins.[16]

Cutaneous pseudolymphoma is a benign but reactive T-cell or B-cell lymphoproliferative disease that often mimics TCRLBCL on histopathology and in humans commonly arises in response to a variety of foreign antigens, including tick bites and *Borrelia burgodorferi* infection.[34] In horses, cutaneous pseudolymphoma has been described in 1 case report[35] and in 1 experimental study, where ponies were treated with dexamethasone and exposed to *Borrelia*-infected *Ixodes* spp. ticks.[36] Whether cutaneous pseudolymphoma due to other causes can occur in horses is unknown; however, if there is uncertainty in the diagnosis or if horses live in a *Borrelia*-endemic area, polymerase chain reaction (PCR) testing of the skin lesion for the organism's DNA and IHC to determine clonality should be pursued.

Treatment

Surgical excision and/or intratumoral therapy, including cytotoxic chemotherapy, are reported treatment options.[4,24,25,27] Intratumoral treatment with cisplatin is a thoroughly described local chemotherapy with only mild local adverse reactions and no systemic toxicities reported.[24] In that report, surgical lesions were treated with cisplatin alone or in combination with surgical debridement.[24] Lyophilized cisplatin was reconstituted with sterile water and mixed with medical-grade sesame oil (60%) and sorbitan monooleate (7%). The solution was injected in 1 or 2 parallel planes, with the goal of infusing 1 mg cisplatin into each cm^3 of tissue.[24]

Systemic lomustine (CCNU) and prednisolone were used successfully in a report due to questionable surgical margins.[30] Importantly, in all cases describing the use of chemotherapeutic agents, adverse reactions were minimal.[4,30] *Borrelia*-associated cutaneous pseudolymphoma can be treated successfully with a 30-day course of doxycycline.[35] If another antigen is suspected, removal of this antigen is reported to resolve the lesion.[34]

Prognosis

Horses with mucocutaneous lymphoma have longer survival times than other anatomic distributions of lymphoma,[4] with a study reporting a median survival of 957 days from diagnosis[16]; another study reported 2 to 5-year survival from the time of first nodule appearance.[37] Recurrence may impact survival in TCRLBCL, with 56% of horses having no recurrence following excision and 83% of horses with no recurrence still alive at follow-up.[25] If local recurrence occurred following surgical excision, survival dropped by 50%.[25] In that study, however, surgical margins, financial constraints, and initial lesion appearance were not assessed, so whether survival was linked solely to recurrence or to other factors is uncertain. In that same study, all horses with CTCL had recurrence, and 33% of the horses were still alive at the time of publication.[25] However, only 3 horses were treated for their CTCL; it is unclear whether that small sample accurately represents a larger population.

A total of 96% of the horses treated with intratumoral cisplatin had a 2-year local control rate independent of tumor size, with tumors less than 2 cm having 100% 2-year local control.[24] Horses treated with chemotherapy in another study had complete remission.[4] The subtype was not reported in either study, so it is unclear whether different subtypes would respond differently to therapy.

ALIMENTARY LYMPHOMA

Alimentary lymphoma is the third most frequent type of lymphoma in horses (behind multicentric and cutaneous),[3] and it is the most frequently diagnosed intestinal neoplasm; in a study, over 56% of the intestinal neoplasia was lymphoma.[19,38] The mean age for alimentary lymphoma ranges from 10 to 16 years of age, but it is notable that this form has been diagnosed in horses 1 year of age[15] and up to 30 years of age.[19]

Pathogenesis

The small intestine is the most frequently affected segment of the gastrointestinal tract, with 2 case series reporting 74%[19] and 60%[15] prevalence. Lymphoma can affect both the small and large colons as well,[12,15,39] with a case series reporting that 47% of horses had both portions affected.[19]

T-cell lymphoma is the predominant sub-type.[12,15,19,39,40] The World Health Organization has classified enteropathy (alimentary)- associated T-cell lymphoma (EATL) into 2 subtypes: EATL and monomorphic epitheliotropic intestinal lymphoma (MEITL), which used to be called EATL2. These 2 entities have been recognized in dogs and cats and have distinct clinical and morphologic features.[41,42] In a case series, horses with T-cell lymphoma were further classified into EATL or MEITL; 40% were found to have EATL, and 45% were found to have MEITL.[15] Importantly, the sub-types carry different prognoses.

In cats and dogs, recent data suggest that inflammatory bowel disease (IBD) in some cases promotes the progression of T-cell lymphoma.[41–44] It is unknown whether IBD could precede the development of T-cell lymphoma in horses. More research and follow-up on cases diagnosed with IBD is required to resolve this question.

Clinical Presentation

Diagnosing alimentary lymphoma antemortem is challenging; a report found that only 38% of cases were diagnosed antemortem.[19] Based on case series and single case reports, the most common clinical signs are poor body condition score,[15,19,39,40,45] loose feces,[15,19,39] fever,[19,46] a history of recurrent colic episodes,[15,19,40,45,47] and ventral edema.[3,19] Most horses in the few available case reports have at least 2 of the aforementioned clinical signs, and the duration of these signs is typically chronic.[19,39,40,46,47]

Diagnostic Testing

The most rewarding diagnostic tests include rectal palpation, transcutaneous abdominal ultrasound, and rectal and/or duodenal biopsies. In some reports, mural thickening of the intestine and/or discrete masses were palpable rectally.[19,39,40] The most common findings on transcutaneous abdominal ultrasound include mural thickening,[12,19] lymphadenopathy,[19,46] or a discrete mass within the alimentary tract.[19,40,46] In a case series, all horses with duodenal (4.5–10 mm) and colonic thickening (4–18 mm) were diagnosed with lymphoma.[19] Abdominocentesis can also be helpful, with a report indicating that 57% of the horses with intestinal neoplasia had increased peritoneal total nucleated cell count (>2000 cells/mL; median total nucleated cell count of 4250 cell/mL, total protein of 2.1 g/dL).[19]

Rectal and duodenal biopsies can detect microscopic abnormalities and, despite representing only a limited portion of the gastrointestinal tract, are often high yield. In a report, rectal biopsies were performed when the clinical suspicion of lymphoma was high, and all biopsies were abnormal.[19] Diagnosis should be possible with histology; however, interobserver variation and ambiguous samples that have features of both inflammatory and neoplastic disease can make histologic diagnosis challenging.[41,48] Based on the literature and author experience, IHC should be pursued on every sample to differentiate cellular infiltrates (T cell vs B cell), to avoid ambiguous interpretation, and to provide prognostic information, as prognosis may vary based on lymphoma subtype.[5,15,16] The American College of Veterinary Internal Medicine (ACVIM) feline consensus statement on differentiation of low-grade neoplastic enteropathies from inflammatory enteropathies has identified IHC as an essential diagnostic tool.[41] Exploratory laparotomy or celiotomy may be helpful, allowing visualization and full-thickness biopsy collection from grossly affected tissue.[12,19] Less invasive techniques should be performed initially, unless the horse is undergoing celiotomy for another reason (eg, acute colic).

Treatment and Prognosis

Treatment options include surgical resection,[12,19] corticosteroids, cytotoxic chemotherapy, or a combination of modalities.[4,15,19,49] There is no "gold standard" for treatment but based on limited case reports and series, systemic immunosuppression likely prolongs survival; prognosis is poor and probably depends on subtype. In a report, survival time of horses treated with systemic chemotherapeutic agents, including corticosteroids, was longer than untreated horses, with the median survival being 151 days and 4 days, respectively.[16] In a case series, lymphoma subtype significantly affected survival, with EATL having a 25-day survival from time of diagnosis, followed by MEITL and TCRLBCL at 90 days and 187.5 days, respectively.[15] Importantly, none of the horses were treated with chemotherapy, and it is not clear which subtype of lymphoma was treated with corticosteroids.[15]

In another case series, treatment of 2 horses with systemic corticosteroids led to euthanasia at 5 months and 1-year post-diagnosis, but their sub-type was not identified.[19] In another study, 3 horses had confirmed alimentary lymphoma; all had a partial response to systemic chemotherapy, and all were euthanized 2, 2.5, and 7 months after diagnosis due to progression of their clinical signs.[4] Unfortunately, it is not clear what the treatment course or lymphoma sub-type was in each case.[4] Based on the literature and the authors' experience, systemic chemotherapy options are detailed in **Table 1**.

ADDITIONAL COMMENTS

More research needs to be done to diagnose equine lymphoma earlier in its clinical course, to develop more accurate antemortem diagnostic tests, and to standardize treatment protocols, with the goal of treatment being accessible, affordable, and effective. If some forms of alimentary lymphoma evolve from IBD, the authors propose close monitoring of horses diagnosed with IBD (including serial rectal biopsies to monitor disease). Additionally, there has been interest surrounding thymidine kinase 1 (TK1) as a diagnostic biomarker for equine lymphoma. In human medicine, it is routinely used as a biomarker for progression, recurrence, and treatment monitoring for a variety of neoplastic conditions.[50,51] Studies in equine lymphoma are conflicting, with a report demonstrating higher serum TK1 activity in horses with multicentric or alimentary lymphoma[52] and another study demonstrating no association with the diagnosis of lymphoma.[14] Interestingly, Moore and colleagues also found no association with fibrinogen or total protein concentrations between horses with lymphoma and those without lymphoma, which differs from other reports.[5,19] It is possible that the utility of serum TK1 activity could depend upon the anatomic location of lymphoma and the duration of disease; however, this requires further exploration.

LEUKEMIA

Leukemia is abnormal proliferation and development of cells within the bone marrow and can be characterized according to the cell of origin (myeloid vs lymphoid), proportion of immature cells, time course of disease (acute or chronic), and the presence of abnormal cells in peripheral circulation. Reported myeloproliferative disorders in horses are malignant histiocytosis, myeloid leukemia, erythroid leukemia, granulocytic leukemia, primary erythrocytosis, and megakaryocytic leukemia. Excluding lymphoma, common lymphoproliferative disorders in horses include lymphoid leukemias and multiple myeloma. For this review, the focus will be on acute versus chronic leukemias since clinical signs and prognosis often depend on this classification and might be more useful to the equine practitioner. Leukemia in horses has been recently reviewed.[53,54]

CLINICAL PRESENTATION
Acute Leukemias

Acute leukemias are generally defined as the presence of immature cells ("blasts") that lack functionality due to their immature status. Whether the leukemia originates from the myeloid or lymphoid lineage, both forms are characterized by rapid disease progression. The most common acute leukemias described in horses are acute myeloid leukemia (AML) and acute lymphoid leukemia (ALL). Horses diagnosed with these conditions tend to be young,[55–58] including 1 report in a 10-week old Thoroughbred filly.[59] In 2 case series, the mean age was 7.2 years with a range of 2 months to 25 years[60]; the mean age was 2.3 years for ALL and 5.3 years for AML.[61] However, older horses can also be diagnosed with acute leukemias and thus, age should not be an exclusion criterion.[60,62]

Clinical signs tend to be acute, ranging from a few days to weeks,[55,56,58,60,61,63] with some case reports reporting multiple months.[57] The most common clinical signs include exercise intolerance, persistent fever, distal limb or ventral edema, weight loss, petechiae, epistaxis, dull mentation, lymphadenopathy, and infections nonresponsive to appropriate antimicrobial therapy.[55–58,60–63]

Chronic Leukemias

Chronic leukemias are generally defined as an inappropriate production of mature cells either from the myeloid or lymphoid lineage. Like acute leukemia, chronic leukemia can originate from the myeloid or lymphoid lineage, and both forms are characterized by relatively slow disease progression. The most common chronic leukemias described in horses are chronic myeloid leukemia (CML) and chronic lymphocytic leukemia (CLL). Information regarding chronic leukemias in horses is scarce and largely derived from case reports.[64–69] Horses diagnosed with chronic leukemias tend to be greater than 14 years old, with 1 report of a 4-year old gelding.[64–69]

Clinical signs tend to be chronic, ranging from 1 month[65] to years,[64] with 1 report of an apparently healthy mare presenting for an annual health check and having only mild generalized peripheral lymphadenopathy.[68] Common clinical signs include edema, persistently enlarged lymph nodes, and exercise intolerance.

DIAGNOSTIC TESTING
Acute Leukemias

Compared with lymphoma, complete blood count is generally rewarding, as common abnormalities include thrombocytopenia, lymphopenia, neutropenia, and/or anemia; most horses present with at least 2 cytopenias.[55–63,70] Importantly, abnormal circulating blood cells (blasts or atypical cells) can be identified[61] but are not always present.[53] The most frequent abnormality on serum biochemical tests is hypoalbuminemia.[58,60,61] A case series found mild increases in serum amyloid A (SAA; 100–650 mg/L) in 4 out of 8 horses and significant increases in SAA (2000–5000 mg/L) in 4 out of 8 horses; however, this was not correlated to clinical presentation, blood work findings, or outcome.[60]

Bone marrow aspirate or biopsy is essential for the diagnosis of acute leukemia and can be performed even in the presence of thrombocytopenia.[55–57,59–62] The most common site is the sternum; although use of the tuber coxae has been reported, it is not recommended.[71] Bone marrow biopsy can reveal the percentage of blasts, cellularity, and the myeloid:erythroid (M:E) ratio of the tumor. Additionally, aspirates of enlarged peripheral lymph nodes can be helpful.

Chronic Leukemia

A complete blood count often reveals persistent leukocytosis, lymphocytosis, and mild anemia,[65–69] and a serum biochemistry can reveal hyperproteinemia.[67–69] In addition to absolute cell counts, blood smears can be helpful to identify abnormal cell morphology.[65,66,68] Serum electrophoresis can discern abnormal serum concentrations of specific immunoglobulins (eg, IgG).[64,67] Bone marrow and lymph node aspirate or biopsy are often helpful to diagnose chronic leukemia and often can confirm clinical suspicion in a horse with persistent leukocytosis.[65–69]

TREATMENT AND PROGNOSIS
Acute Leukemia

Based on limited case reports and series, the prognosis for acute leukemia is grave, with most horses being euthanized within 3 days of diagnosis due to rapidly progressive clinical signs.[55,59–61,70] Unlike lymphoma, the prognosis for acute leukemia does not appear to improve with the administration of systemic glucocorticoids or chemotherapy. In a case report, 3 out of 6 horses with AML and 2 out of 6 with ALL were treated with systemic corticosteroids but were euthanized 1 to 7 days and 3 and 42 days after diagnosis, respectively, due to deterioration of clinical signs.[60] In another case report, a horse diagnosed with AML was treated with prednisolone once a day for 11 days before being euthanized for progressive weight loss, epistaxis, and hematuria.[62] Systemic chemotherapy had been attempted with vincristine, cytarabine, and prednisone, but the horse was euthanized 3 days later.[61] The rapid disease progression of acute leukemias likely is one reason treatment is unsuccessful and the prognosis is grave. In human medicine, treatment of acute leukemias often relies on a combination of chemotherapy, allogeneic hematopoietic stem cell transplantation (alloHSCT), and novel therapeutics (eg, monoclonal antibodies and specific small molecule inhibitors).[72,73] In horses, alloHSCT has not been attempted, and the use of novel therapies is limited due to the lack of genetic testing and cost. Therefore, achieving a level of therapeutic precision in horses that might be required to successfully treat acute leukemias will likely remain challenging for the foreseeable future.

Chronic Leukemia

Due to the slow progression of the disease, chronic leukemias appear to have a more favorable prognosis; however, given the scarcity of published reports, this is largely speculation. In a report, both horses received no treatment and were euthanized approximately 2.5 and 4.5 months following initial diagnosis, but both horses had clinical signs before diagnosis for 24 months and 7 months, respectively.[64] In another case report, a horse with enlarged lymph nodes received no treatment and was euthanized 2 months later for dysphagia secondary to lymphadenopathy.[67] One horse presented for a routine physical examination was diagnosed with CLL, received no treatment, and remained clinically stable for 120 days, at which point a marked leukocytosis developed; the horse was euthanized 194 days after initial diagnosis for lethargy and dyspnea.[68]

It is unclear whether systemic immunosuppressive therapy would improve the outcome of horses with chronic leukemia. In a case with B-cell CLL, the horse was treated with prednisolone for 1 week and then chlorambucil.[65] In this report, there was an initial decrease in lymphocyte count after the first dose of chlorambucil; however, after the second dose of chlorambucil, the lymphocyte counts increased, and the horse became persistently febrile weeks after chlorambucil was discontinued and was euthanized 6 weeks after initial presentation to the hospital.[65] In a case series, 3 horses received oral corticosteroids with survival following diagnosis being 12 months, 11 months, and 3 days.[69] In the same case series, a horse received no treatment and survived 5 years following diagnosis, while 3 other horses received no treatment and died weeks later.[69] Based on these limited reports, the impact of immunosuppressive therapy could depend on the subtype of chronic leukemia and the duration of the disease prior to diagnosis.

SUMMARY

Lymphoma and myeloproliferative diseases in horses are relatively uncommon. The clinical signs, prognosis, and treatment options depend upon the anatomic location and subtype. Significant gaps in knowledge remain regarding prevalence, pathogenesis of different sub-types, antemortem diagnostic tests, response to treatment, and standardized treatment protocols. However, treatment options are available, accessible on the farm, and could improve quality of life and prolong survival.

CLINICS CARE POINTS

- When administering cytotoxic chemotherapy IV, a dedicated IV catheter placed with a single, clean venipuncture should be used; ideally, a new catheter should be placed for each dose. Application of topical diclofenac cream (Surpass™, Boehringer-Ingelheim) and/or DMSO gel, along with hot compress application, can be helpful for minimizing phlebitis between treatments.

- Partnering with a human hospital can be helpful for disposing of biomedical waste associated with on-farm cytotoxic chemotherapy administration.

- Monitoring size of lesions with calipers and/or ultrasonography, along with serial hemograms, is helpful for assessing response to treatment.

- In horses receiving treatment for lymphoma or leukemia, modification of the diet may be helpful to minimize weight loss (increased fat and fiber, rotating palatable feedstuffs, flavoring agents) and risk of serious complications of prolonged corticosteroid use, such as laminitis (minimize dietary non-structural carbohydrate content of the diet, ideally <10% on a dry matter basis).

DISCLOSURE

The authors declare no conflict of interest.

REFERENCES

1. Miller MA, Moore GE, Bertin FR, et al. What's new in old horses? postmortem diagnoses in mature and aged equids. Vet Pathol 2016;53:390–8.
2. Knowles EJ, Tremaine WH, Pearson GR, et al. A database survey of equine tumours in the United Kingdom. Equine Vet J 2016;48:280–4.
3. Durham AC, Pillitteri CA, San Myint M, et al. Two hundred three cases of equine lymphoma classified According to the World Health Organization (WHO) Classification Criteria. Vet Pathol 2012;50:86–93.
4. Luethy D, Frimberger AE, Bedenice D, et al. Retrospective evaluation of clinical outcome after chemotherapy for lymphoma in 15 equids (1991-2017). J Vet Intern Med 2019;33:953–60.
5. Meyer J, DeLay J, Bienzle D. Clinical, laboratory, and histopathologic features of equine lymphoma. Vet Pathol 2006;43:914–24.
6. Mair TS, Brown PJ. Clinical and pathological features of thoracic neoplasia in the horse. Equine Vet J 1993;25:220–3.
7. Torrent A, Kilcoyne I, Johnson A, et al. Case Report: An atypical presentation of multi-systemic B-cell lymphoma in a horse. Can Vet J 2019;60:300–4.
8. Sano Y, Okamoto M, Ootsuka Y, et al. Blindness associated with nasal/paranasal lymphoma in a stallion. J Vet Med Sci 2017;79:579–83.
9. Gillen A, Mudge M, Caldwell F, et al. Outcome of external beam radiotherapy for treatment of noncutaneous tumors of the head in horses: 32 cases (1999-2015). J Vet Intern Med 2020;34:2808–16.
10. Montgomery JB, Duckett WM, Bourque AC. Pelvic lymphoma as a cause of urethral compression in a mare. Can Vet J 2009;50:751–4.
11. Sweeney RW, Hamir AN, Fisher RR. Lymphosarcoma with urinary bladder infiltration in a horse. J Am Vet Med Assoc 1991;199:1177–8.
12. Miglio A, Morelli C, Gialletti R, et al. Clinical and immunophenotypic findings in 4 forms of equine lymphoma. Can Vet J 2019;60:33–40.
13. Taylor SD, Haldorson GJ, Vaughan B, et al. Gastric neoplasia in horses. J Vet Intern Med 2009;23:1097–102.
14. Moore C, Stefanovski D, Luethy D. Clinical performance of a commercially available thymidine kinase 1 assay for diagnosis of lymphoma in 42 hospitalized horses (2017-2020). J Vet Intern Med 2021;35:2495–9.
15. Bacci B, Stent AW, Walmsley EA. Equine intestinal lymphoma: clinical-pathological features, immunophenotype, and survival. Vet Pathol 2020;57: 369–76.
16. Wensley FM, Berryhill EH, Magdesian GK. Association of globulin concentrations with prognosis in horses with lymphoma. Front Vet Sci 2023;9:1–12.
17. Roccabianca P, Paltrinieri S, Gallo E, et al. Hepatosplenic T-cell Lymphoma in a Mare. Vet Pathol 2002;39:508–11.
18. Kelton DR, Holbrook TC, Gilliam LL, et al. Bone marrow necrosis and myelophthisis: Manifestations of T-cell lymphoma in a horse. Vet Clin Pathol 2008;37:403–8.
19. Taylor SD, Pusterla N, Vaughan B, et al. Intestinal Neoplasia in Horses. J Vet Intern Med 2006;20:1429–36.
20. Neufeld JL. Lymphosarcoma in a mare and review of cases at the ontario veterinary college. Can Vet J 1973;14:1–5.
21. Canisso I, Pinn TL, Gerdin J, et al. B-cell multicentric lymphoma as a probably cause of abortion in a Quarter horse broodmare. Can Vet J 2013;54:288–91.
22. Valentine BA. Survey of equine cutaneous neoplasia in the Pacific Northwest. J Vet Diagn Invest 2006;18:123–6.

23. Schaffer PA, Wobeser B, Martin LER, et al. Cutaneous neoplastic lesions of equids in the central United States and Canada: 3,351 biopsy specimens from 3,272 equids (2000-2010). J Am Vet Med Assoc 2013;242:99–105.

24. Theon AP, Wilson DW, Magdesian GK, et al. Long-term outcome associated with intratumor chemotherapy with cisplatin for cutaneous tumors in equidae: 573 cases (1995-2004). J Am Vet Med Assoc 2007;230:1506–14.

25. Miller CA, Durham AC, Schaffer PA, et al. Classification and clinical features in 88 cases of equine cutaneous lymphoma. J Vet Diagn Invest 2015;27:86–91.

26. Kelley LC, Mahaffey EA. Equine malignant lymphomas: morphologic and immunohistochemical classification. Vet Pathol 1998;35:241–52.

27. Littlewood JD, Whitwell KE, Day MJ. Equine cutaneous lymphoma: a case report. Vet Dermatol 1995;6:105–11.

28. Johnson PJ. Dermatologic Tumors (excluding sarcoids). Vet Clin N Am Equine Pract 1998;14:625–58.

29. Epstein V, Hodge D. Cutaneous lymphosarcoma in a stallion. Aust Vet J 2005;83: 609–11.

30. Doyle AJ, Macdonald VS, Bourque A. Use of lomustine (CCNU) in a case of cutaneous equine lymphoma. Can Vet J 2013;54:1137–42.

31. Henker LC, Dal Pont TP, Santos IR, et al. Pathology in Practice. J Am Vet Med Assoc 2021;259(S2).

32. Henson KL, Alleman AR, Cutler TJ, et al. Regression of subcutaneous lymphoma following removal of an ovarian granulosatheca cell tumor in a horse. J Am Vet Med Assoc 1998;212:419–22.

33. Henson KL, Alleman AR, Kelley LC, et al. Immunohistochemical characterization of estrogen and progesterone receptors in lymphoma of horses. Vet Clin Pathol 2000;29:40–6.

34. Bergman R. Pseudolymphoma and cutaneous lymphoma: Facts and controversies. Clin Dermatol 2010;28:568–74.

35. Sears KP, Divers TJ, Neff RT, et al. A case of Borrelia-associated cutaneous pseudolymphoma in a horse. Vet Dermatol 2012;23:153–6.

36. Chang YF, Novosol V, McDonough SP, et al. Experimental infection of ponies with borrelia burgdorferi by exposure to ixodid ticks. Vet Pathol 2000;37:68–76.

37. de Bruijn CM, Veenman JN, Rutten VPMG, et al. Clinical, histopathological and immunophenotypical findings in five horses with cutaneous malignant lymphoma. Res Vet Sci 2007;83:63–72.

38. Baker JR, Ellis CE. A survey of post mortem findings in 480 horses 1958 to 1980: (1) Causes of death. Equine Vet J 1981;13:43–6.

39. Sanz MG, Sellon DC, Potter KA. Primary epitheliotropic intestinal T-cell lymphoma as a cause of diarrhea in a horse. Can Vet J 2010;51:522–4.

40. Sherlock C, Dawson L, Mair T. Ultrasound as a diagnostic tool in the investigation of a pony with intestinal lymphoma. Equine Vet Educ 2017;29:78–81.

41. Marsilio S, Freiche V, Johnson E, et al. ACVIM consensus statement guidelines on diagnosing and distinguishing low-grade neoplastic from inflammatory lymphocytic chronic enteropathies in cats. J Vet Intern Med 2023;37:794–816.

42. Matsumoto I, Nakashima K, Goto-Koshino Y, et al. Immunohistochemical profiling of canine intestinal t-cell lymphomas. Vet Pathol 2019;56(1):50–60.

43. Sabattini S, Bottero E, Turba ME, et al. Differentiating feline inflammatory bowel disease from alimentary lymphoma in duodenal endoscopic biopsies. J Small Anim Pract 2016;57:396–401.

44. Wright KZ, Hohenhaus AE, Verrilli AM, et al. Feline large-cell lymphoma following previous treatment for small-cell gastrointestinal lymphoma: incidence, clinical

signs, clinicopathologic data, treatment of a secondary malignancy, response and survival. J Feline Med Surg 2019;21:353–62.

45. Hillyer MH, Mair TS. Recurrent colic in the mature horse: A retrospective review of 58 cases. Equine Vet J 1997;29:421–4.

46. Acevedo HD, Hassebroek AM, Leventhal HR, et al. Colonic T-cell-rich, large B-cell lymphoma associated with equid herpesvirus 5 infection and secondary trans-colonic fistula in a horse. J Vet Diagn Invest 2023;35:272–7.

47. Platt BH. Alimentary lymphomas in the horse. J Comp Pathol 1987;97:1–10.

48. Willard MD, Jergens AE, Duncan RB, et al. Interobserver variation among histopathologic evaluations of intestinal tissues from dogs and cats. J Am Vet Med Assoc 2002;220:1177–83.

49. Byrne BA, Yvorchuk-St-Jean K, Couto CG, et al. Successful management of lymphoproliferative disease in two pregnant mares. In: Proceedings of the 11th Annual Conference Veterinary Cancer Society; Fort Collins, CO, USA, October 27-29, 1991; 1991:8-9.

50. Bitter EE, Townsend MH, Erickson R, et al. Thymidine kinase 1 through the ages: a comprehensive review. Cell Biosci 2020;10:1–16.

51. Fanelli GN, Scarpitta R, Cinacchi P, et al. Immunohistochemistry for thymidine kinase-1 (Tk1): A potential tool for the prognostic stratification of breast cancer patients. J Clin Med 2021;10:1–13.

52. Wang L, Unger L, Sharif H, et al. Molecular characterization of equine thymidine kinase 1 and preliminary evaluation of its suitability as a serum biomarker for equine lymphoma. BMC Mol Cell Biol 2021;22:1–12.

53. Satué K, Gardon JC, Muñoz A. A review of current knowledge of myeloproliferative disorders in the horse. Acta Vet Scand 2021;63(1):1–11.

54. Muñoz A, Riber C, Trigo P, et al. Hematopoietic neoplasias in horses: myeloproliferative and lymphoproliferative disorders. J Equine Sci 2009;20:59–72.

55. Lester GD, Alleman AR, Raskin RE, et al. Pancytopenia secondary to lymphoid leukemia in three horses. J Vet Intern Med 1993;7:360–3.

56. Ringger NC, Edens L, Bain P, et al. Acute myelogenous leukaemia in a mare. Aust Vet J 1997;75:329–31.

57. Miglio A, Pepe M, Felippe MJB, et al. Subleukaemic acute myeloid leukaemia with myelodysplasia in a horse. Equine Vet Educ 2019;31:e39–46.

58. Furness MC, Setlakwe E, Sallaway J, et al. Acute myeloid leukemia with basophilic differentiation in a 3-year-old Standardbred gelding. Can Vet J 2016;57: 1067–71.

59. Forbes G, Feary DJ, Savage CJ, et al. Acute myeloid leukaemia (M6B: Pure acute erythroid leukaemia) in a Thoroughbred foal. Aust Vet J 2011;89:269–72.

60. Cooper CJ, Keller SM, Arroyo LG, et al. Acute leukemia in horses. Vet Pathol 2018;55:159–72.

61. Barrell EA, Asakawa MG, Felippe MJB, et al. Acute leukemia in six horses (1990–2012). J Vet Diagn Invest 2017;29(4):529–35.

62. Clark P, Cornelisse CJ, Schott HC, et al. Myeloblastic leukaemia in a Morgan horse mare. Equine Vet J 1999;31:446–8.

63. Bienzle D, Hughson SL, Vernau W. Acute myelomonocytic leukemia in a horse. Can Vet J 1993;34:36–7.

64. Trenton McClure J, Young KM, Fiste M, et al. Immunophenotypic classification of leukemia in 3 horses. J Vet Intern Med 2001;15:144–52.

65. Long AE, Javsicas LH, Stokol T, et al. Rapid clinical progression of B-cell chronic lymphocytic leukemia in a horse. J Am Vet Med Assoc 2019;255:716–22.

66. Johansson AM, Skidell J, Lilliehook I, et al. Chronic granulocytic leukemia in a horse. J Am Vet Med Assoc 2007;21:1126–9.

67. Dascanio JJ, Zhang CH, Antczak DF, et al. Differentiation of chronic lymphocytic leukemia in the horse: a report of two cases. J Vet Intern Med 1992;6:225–9.

68. Cian F, Tyner G, Martini V, et al. Leukemic small cell lymphoma or chronic lymphocytic leukemia in a horse. Vet Clin Pathol 2013;42:301–6.

69. Rendle DI, Durham AE, Thompson JC, et al. Clinical, immunophenotypic and functional characterisation of T-cell leukaemia in six horses. Equine Vet J 2007; 39:522–8.

70. Buechner-Maxwell V, Zhang C, Robertson J, et al. Intravascular leukostasis and systemic aspergillosis in a horse with subleukemic acute myelomonocytic leukemia. J Vet Intern Med 1994;8:258–63.

71. Delling U, Linder K, Ribitsch I, et al. Comparison of bone marrow aspiration at the sternum and tuber coxae in middle-aged horses. Can J Vet Res 2012;76:52–6.

72. Shimony S, Stahl M, Stone RM. Acute myeloid leukemia: 2023 update on diagnosis, risk-stratification, and management. Am J Hematol 2023;98:502–26.

73. Rafei H, Kantarjian HM, Jabbour EJ. Recent advances in the treatment of acute lymphoblastic leukemia. Leuk Lymphoma 2019;60:2606–21.

74. Burns T, Couto G. Systemic chemotherapy for oncologic diseases. In: Robinson N, Sprayberry K, editors. Current therapy in equine medicine. 6th edition. St. Louis, MO: Saunders; 2009. p. 15–8.

75. Théon AP, Pusterla N, Magdesian KG, et al. A pilot phase II study of the efficacy and biosafety of doxorubicin chemotherapy in tumor-bearing equidae. J Vet Intern Med 2013;27:1581–8.

76. Théon AP, Pusterla N, Magdesian KG, et al. Phase I dose escalation of doxorubicin chemotherapy in tumor-bearing equidae. J Vet Intern Med 2013;27: 1209–17.

Oral and Sinonasal Tumors

Padraic M. Dixon, MVB, PhD, FRCVS

KEYWORDS

- Equine oral tumors • Equine sinonasal tumors • Equine tumors

KEY POINTS

- Tumors and non-neoplastic growths of the equine oral cavity appear uncommon compared with some other domestic animal species.
- Oral squamous cell carcinomas are aggressive, often very extensive when diagnosed and so carry a poor prognosis.
- Juvenile ossifying fibromas of the rostral jaws are a characteristic growth of young horses that also carry a good prognosis following resection.
- Non-neoplastic sinonasal growths are 2 to 3 times more prevalent than sinonasal neoplasms.
- Soft tissue sinonasal neoplasms, such as squamous cell carcinomas or adenocarcinomas, carry a poor prognosis in contrast to calcified bone or dental tumors.

ORAL TUMORS

Introduction

Oral neoplasia is uncommon in horses, with less than 1.1% of equine neoplasms reported to develop directly in the mouth.[1,2] Many equine practitioners may never recognize such lesions during their careers.[3] The relative shortage of reported series of equine oral neoplastic and nonneoplastic growths (such as gingival hyperplasia) also suggests that these lesions are rare. However, no significant studies have been reported that classified and quantified equine oral tumors using larger multicenter studies, which are necessary because of the apparent scarcity of these lesions.[4] Meanwhile, smaller case series[3,5] and even single case reports of unusual equine oral growths remain of value owing to the paucity of literature on these lesions.

The gross appearance of some oral neoplasms and non-neoplastic growths can be similar (eg, odontogenic tumors and bone cysts both cause localized, painless jaw swellings), and histology is usually required to make a definitive diagnosis. A description of the main non-neoplastic oral growths is therefore initially given to aid their recognition. Most equine oral neoplasms are malignant, with squamous cell carcinomas (SCCs) being the most common of these lesions. Only small numbers of benign

9 Durham Road, Edinburgh, EH15 1NU, UK
E-mail address: padraicdixon@outlook.com

Vet Clin Equine 40 (2024) 455–473
https://doi.org/10.1016/j.cveq.2024.07.010
0749-0739/24/© 2024 Elsevier Inc. All rights reserved, including those for text and data mining, AI training, and similar technologies.

vetequine.theclinics.com

equine oral neoplasms have been reported.[6] Odontogenic tumors are usually benign but are expansive and can be locally destructive within the jaws, whereas SCCs are usually well-advanced with much local infiltration before they are diagnosed, and therefore, difficult to effectively treat. The rostral mandibular area is more prone to develop neoplasia than the mid or caudal mandible.[7]

Using a pathologist who specializes in oral pathology can significantly improve the accuracy of diagnosis because many of these tumors are very rare, and pathologists may only see a handful of them in their lifetime.[6] In addition, the histopathological interpretation of some of these lesions, especially of fibro-osseous lesions, is not always definitive. Evaluation of the history, clinical signs, and diagnostic images can help the pathologist develop a more complete clinical picture and reach a pathological diagnosis that best represents the examined lesions.[6] This article is primarily directed to help the equine practitioner diagnose and prognosticate on equine oral tumors. For further pathological information and more extensive bibliographies on these growths, the reader is referred to the excellent texts by Knottenbelt and colleagues,[4] and in particular, to the pathological descriptions of oral tumors by Bienert-Zeit and colleagues.[6]

Oral tumors can potentially involve every cell type that occurs in the oral cavity, but this review only deals with specific oral tumors, such as odontogenic (dental) tumors and the more commonly recorded other types of tumors. The section is divided into 4 categories, as shown below.

Categories of Oral Tumors
  Nonneoplastic growths
  Soft tissue tumors
  Odontogenic tumors
  Bone tumors

ORAL NON-NEOPLASTIC GROWTHS

  Nodular hypercementosis (cemental hyperplasia, "cement pearls")
  Fibrous and gingival hyperplasia
  Aneurysmal and solitary bone cysts
  Periapical (radicular) cysts
  Hamartomas
  Eruption "cysts"

Nodular Hypercementosis

Nodular hypercementosis (reactive hypercementosis, "cemental pearls") are reactive, non-neoplastic cemental masses that are often incorrectly termed "cementomas." These nodular hypercementosis lesions may be multiple and most commonly occur at periapical infections or post-extraction sites (**Fig. 1**). They are seldom greater than 20 mm in diameter, unlike cementomas, which are usually much larger. The author does not consider nodular hypercementosis to be clinically significant in most cases and does not usually curette them unless they are readily accessible in the alveolus of extracted teeth.

Gingival Hyperplasia

Gingival hyperplasia are fleshy lesions that appear along the gingival margins and are usually flat (<20 mm deep) and may extend along the margins of many teeth. The

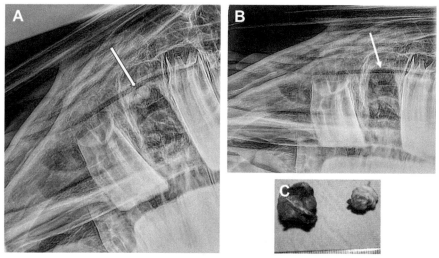

Fig. 1. (*A*) Radiograph of a 207 extraction site containing radiodense, rounded structures at its apex (*arrows*), that is, nodular hypercementosis lesions ("cement(al) pearls"). (*B*) This radiograph was obtained after two such lesions (*C*) were curetted from the alveolus.

underlying bones appear normal. Under local anesthesia, the lesions can be elevated and resected with margins and histopathology performed (**Fig. 2**). Another benign gingival lesion is a fibromatous epulis (**Fig. 3**).

Bone Cysts

A bone cyst is defined as a benign, intraosseous fluid-filled expansion surrounded by a thin wall of bone. Bone cysts include extensive blood-filled and often destructive aneurysmal bone cysts (possibly owing to vascular anomalies) or less destructive, solitary bone cysts. The latter could be clinically mistaken for intraosseous tumors, but bone cysts have characteristic imaging appearances. They are treated by curettage of the cyst lining.

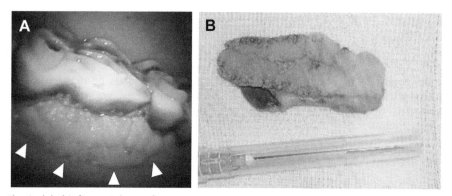

Fig. 2. (*A*) This firm painless, soft tissue growth lying below the gingival margin of 407 and 408 (outlined by *arrowheads*) was detected at a routine dental examination. (*B*) Following its excision under local anesthesia, histopathology showed it to be fibrous gingival hyperplasia.

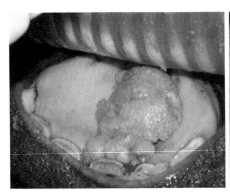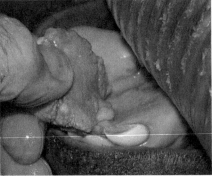

Fig. 3. This pedunculated fibromatous epulis (peripheral odontogenic fibroma) was found at a routine dental examination in a horse without clinical signs.

Eruption "Cysts"

The long (hypsodont) equine teeth (especially in ponies) can become vertically impacted during eruption and thus cause pressure changes and remodeling of the alveolar and supporting bones beneath their apices. These swellings are commonly but erroneously termed eruption "cysts." These painless and bilateral swellings, that do not have a cyst lining, appear on the ventral aspect of the mandible beneath the erupting Triadan 07 and 08 teeth, usually at 3 to 5 years of age. They occur less noticeably as maxillary swellings just rostrodorsal to the rostral aspect of the facial crest. These swellings invariably self-resolve within a couple of years as the supporting bones elongate in a rostrocaudal direction and allow the impacted teeth to normally erupt.

Radicular (Periapical; Root) Cysts

Radicular (periapical; root) cysts are rare in horses compared with small animals. These cysts develop from residual embryologic ectodermal tissue in the periodontium, often at an infected tooth apex. They slowly expand causing root resorption and a firm, localized painless apical swelling. Imaging shows a cystic structure adjacent to an inflamed dental apex with pressure changes on the adjacent bone. Treatment is by exodontia of the affected tooth, and resection of the cyst and carries an excellent prognosis.

Hamartomas

Hamartomas are non-neoplastic growths composed of tissues normally found at that particular site but arranged in an abnormal manner and so can resemble a neoplasm. Some equine osteomas and cementomas can be classified as hamartomas.

ORAL EPITHELIAL NEOPLASMS

Squamous cell carcinoma
Fibroma and fibrosarcoma
Fibro-osseous (ossifying fibroma) tumors such as juvenile ossifying fibroma
Nonspecific tumors, for example, lymphosarcoma, hemangioma, and melanoma

Oral Squamous Cell Carcinoma

SCC is the most common oral neoplasia of horses (see also article "Squamous Cell Carcinomas in Horses: An Update of the Etiopathogenesis and Treatment Options" in this textbook) and more commonly occurs at other sites, including the third eyelid, male genitalia, stomach, and pharynx. It is a highly invasive, squamous epithelium neoplasm that usually develops on the equine oral mucosa and gingiva, or rarely on the tongue epithelium. It has a predilection to develop at mucosal junctions.[6] The author has most commonly recorded SCCs developing in the mucosa or gingiva at the palatal aspect of the caudal maxillary cheek teeth. It has been suggested that SCC may arise at sites of chronic inflammation, such as periodontitis, but the caudal maxillary interdental spaces are an uncommon site of periodontal disease. Oral SCCs have also been associated with different *Equus caballus* papillomaviruses.[6]

Clinical Signs

Cases of oral SCC may initially present with oral malodor because of secondary infection of locally invaded tissues and of the fast-growing tumor. Most cases develop facial swelling (**Figs. 4** and **5**) soon after tumor recognition along with possible dysphagia and weight loss. SCCs that develop on the maxillary oral epithelium may invade dorsally into the paranasal sinuses, causing ipsilateral nasal purulent discharge. Because many oral SCC tumors develop in the caudal oral cavity, they are usually well advanced before facial swelling occurs.

Oral examination shows a large, ulcerated, red fleshy growth protruding from the oral mucosa with extensive invasion of adjacent soft and bony tissues (see **Figs. 4** and **5**) and possibly displaced or loose teeth. Swollen ipsilateral submandibular lymph nodes are invariably present and usually caused by inflammation and secondary infection around the tumor. Lymph node metastases can occur, but distant metastasis is rare. Pharyngeal SCC lesions can also cause dysphagia, malodorous breath, and weight loss.

Diagnosis

Oral SCCs must be differentiated from noncalcified neoplastic or non-neoplastic growths. Deep infected oral wounds or oral foreign body damage may cause a similar

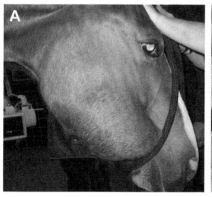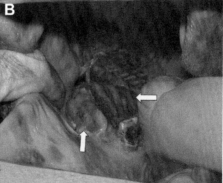

Fig. 4. (*A*) This horse presented with a very rapidly growing swelling of its right mandibular region. (*B*) Oral examination showed an ulcerated, fleshy growth lying buccal to the right mandibular cheek teeth that extended the full length of the oral cavity (*arrows*). It was readily biopsied and found to be an SCC.

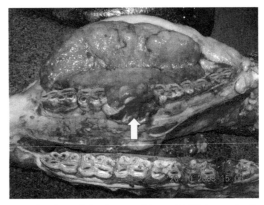

Fig. 5. Postmortem examination of the horse with oral SCC shown in **Fig. 4** shows a massive soft tissue tumor of the right mandible with expansion of the bone and loss of the Triadan 408 tooth (*arrow*).

appearance. It is relatively easy to obtain a large, deep biopsy beneath any necrotic surface and allow a definitive histological diagnosis. Radiography may show bone destruction, but computed tomographic (CT) examination allows exact determination of tumor extension and aggressiveness of oral neoplasms[5] as is also the case with sinonasal neoplasms.[8]

Treatment and Prognosis

Because of extensive local and regional invasion and their common caudal oral location, surgical excision (see article "Surgical Management of Equine Neoplasia") is often impossible by the time of diagnosis, and in any case, is usually unsuccessful. If detected early, especially if located in the rostral oral cavity, complete surgical excision may be possible. Intralesional injections with cisplatin or 5-fluorouracil, or radiotherapy are other possible treatments that are described elsewhere in this publication (see articles "Chemotherapeutics in Equine Practice" and "Radiotherapy in Equine Practice") but usually carry a poor prognosis.

Oral Fibroma/Fibrosarcoma

Fibromas are slow-growing benign fibrous tissue neoplasms. Fibrosarcomas are the malignant variant, although they are also usually slow-growing. These tumors develop from fibrous cells in the subcutaneous tissues, gingival margins, or periosteum, with fibrosarcomas derived from the latter tissues termed periosteal fibrosarcomas.[4] They are considered rare by many investigators,[4,6] although some earlier literature described them as being the second most common oral neoplasm, after SCC.

Clinical features

Oral fibrosarcomas present as red fleshy, local protruding growths on the oral mucosa or gingival margins (**Fig. 6**) with no changes in the underlying bones (unless it is a periosteal fibrosarcoma). These lesions may be locally invasive with rare metastases. Lesions may initially resemble an early SCC or benign gingival hyperplasia.

Diagnosis

Because the clinical appearance is similar to other soft tissue oral lesions, histopathology of a biopsy or of the excised lesion is required. Fibrosarcomas may be well-differentiated and histologically similar to granulation or scar tissue.[9]

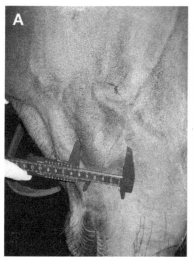
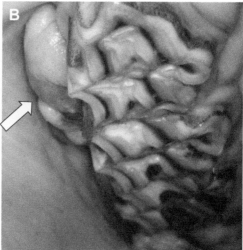

Fig. 6. (*A*) This horse has a 5-cm-diameter firm swelling of its right maxillary gingival region that protrudes through the cheeks. (*B*) An intraoral image of an ulcerated, fleshy growth attached to the buccal gingiva (*arrow*) that was histologically shown to be a fibrosarcoma.

Treatment and prognosis

Small fibrosarcomas with identifiable margins can be surgically resected if accessible (ie, if located in the rostral oral cavity) but can recur, and the prognosis is guarded.[4,6] Horbal and Dixon[9] described a fibrosarcoma on the rostral maxillary buccal-gingival margin (see **Fig. 6**) that was repeatedly treated with intralesional cisplatin injections and surgical resections, and eventually responded to these treatments, with a follow-up of 5 years.

Juvenile Ossifying Fibroma

A juvenile ossifying fibroma is a benign, fast-growing, locally aggressive fibro-osseous neoplasia of young horses (usually <1 year old) that can cause much local damage to the rostral mandible and less commonly to the rostral aspect of the incisive bones, but do not metastasize.[6]

Clinical features

Juvenile ossifying fibromas have a near-pathognomonic appearance (**Fig. 7**) and rapidly develop over a period of a few weeks within the rostral mandible or incisive bones, causing thickening and local disruption of the affected area, and possibly loosening of the adjacent incisor teeth. Typically, a nonpainful golf ball–sized (or larger) mass protrudes through the bone by the time of referral. Lesions initially are covered with intact mucosa that later becomes ulcerated. Most lesions are firm and painless but occasionally can be fleshy. They seldom interfere with prehension, or nursing, and the young horses remain healthy and in good body condition.

Diagnosis

The clinical appearance along with the young age is very diagnostic, but an ameloblastoma, or rostral jaw trauma with granulation tissue,[10] can have a similar appearance. Imaging can help determine the margins of the tumor, and slower-growing lesions (rare) may be calcified and radiographically resemble an osteoma.[6] Histology is

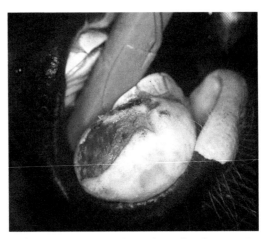

Fig. 7. A 6-month-old foal is under general anesthesia for the resection of a large juvenile ossifying fibroma involving most of its rostral mandible.

necessary for confirmation and is best performed on the excised lesions to limit further spread of the lesion while awaiting histopathologic confirmation.

Treatment and prognosis

These tumors should be surgically excised as soon as possible to allow minimal resection of mandibular or incisive bones. If lesions are longstanding (immature horses do not have regular oral inspections unlike ridden horses), they may involve the caudal aspect of the mandibular symphysis, and such cases need mandibular stabilization after rostral mandibulectomy. The author is conservative with resection, removing just a few millimeters of normal-appearing tissue caudal or medial to the obvious lesion. The lesions can be readily reexamined about 4 weeks postoperatively, and any suspect areas of regrowth can be curetted under sedation and local anesthesia (but is seldom necessary). The prognosis is excellent, but cases should be monitored for possible regrowth, and suspect areas curetted with histopathology of excised tissue performed.

Oral Melanoma

Melanomas are usually found in grey horses (see article "Equine Melanoma Updates" in this textbook) and can develop in the lips and present as discrete spherical, or more diffuse slow-growing, firm, painless lesions. They can also occur in the oral cavity where they may appear as dark submucosal growths. These oral melanomas are usually accompanied by melanomas at the more typical perineal, parotid, and submucosal guttural pouch sites. Oral melanomas are sometimes detected incidentally at dental examinations of grey horses where they rarely cause clinical signs.

Diagnosis

These lesions can usually be diagnosed on clinical examination or at surgery where deeper lesions have the near-pathognomonic appearance of black, homogenous soft tissue.

Treatment and prognosis

Lip lesions are best treated by excisional surgery with margins, and lesions are readily identified to allow such margins. The surgical site in the very mobile lips should be meticulously repaired. Intralesional cisplatin should be administered with great care at this site (as in nonpedunculated lesions at other sites) in case the complex lip musculature is excessively damaged.

ODONTOGENIC (DENTAL) TUMORS

Ameloblastoma/ameloblastic carcinoma
Compound odontoma
Complex odontoma
Cementoma

Equine dental tumors are rare yet may be more common in horses than in other domestic species.[4] They are histologically classified by their tissue of origin, that is, ectodermal epithelium (ameloblasts), ectomesenchymal cells (odontoblasts), or mesenchymal cells of the dental follicle (cementoblasts). They are further classified by the inductive effects of these cells on each other, that is, ameloblasts cannot form calcified enamel unless induced by odontoblasts. Likewise, odontoblasts cannot produce calcified dentine unless induced by ameloblasts. Dental tumors develop within the alveoli and are usually slow-growing and benign but cause local destruction by expanding within the alveoli and causing jaw swellings.

Dental tumors can include ectodermal tumors (derived from the epithelium that forms enamel) termed ameloblastomas. The enamel in these tumors remains noncalcified; however, ameloblastomas may have some diffuse calcification.[5] Dental tumors also include calcified tumors of dentinal origin (odontomas), of cementum (cementomas), or combinations of enamel and dentine (compound and complex odontomas).

Ameloblastoma and Ameloblastic Carcinoma

Ameloblastomas are benign tumors of odontogenic epithelium that have differentiated into ameloblasts but without calcified enamel formation, and ameloblastic carcinomas are their malignant forms.[5,6] Although rare, ameloblastomas may occur more frequently in horses than in other domestic animals.[4] Morgan and colleagues[5] found these to be the most common odontogenic equine tumor comprising 9 out of 11 cases of odontogenic tumors and included a subgroup of 3 nonmineralized ameloblastic fibromas.

Clinical features

Ameloblastomas, as noted, develop within the mandibular or maxillary alveoli causing firm, localized, nonpainful jaw swellings (**Fig. 8**). Soft tissue swellings may eventually protrude through the expanded bone. These *intraosseous* dental tumors can be differentiated from SCC and fibrosarcoma that overlie these bones.

Diagnosis

Imaging will show an expansile mass within the jaws (**Fig. 9**) that may have mineral attenuation.[5] The lesion may be somewhat loculated (often more bone destruction is present), resembling a localized aneurysmal bone cyst; histopathology is essential for confirmation and can be performed on the surgically excised tumor.

Treatment and prognosis

Treatment is by complete surgical excision of early or smaller lesions, along with resection of the supporting bones if ameloblastic carcinomas are present. Intralesional chemotherapy is possible as is radiotherapy in some facilities.[11,12] The prognosis is good if tumors can be fully excised with margins.

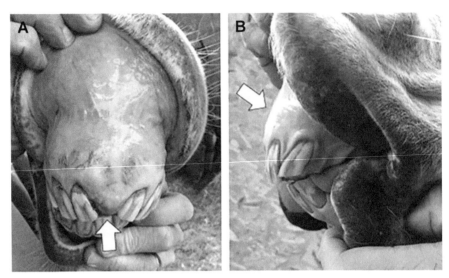

Fig. 8. (*A*) A 12-year-old Connemara pony with recent prehension problems was found to have distal (lateral) incisor displacements causing a diastema between 101 and 201 (*arrow*) and (*B*) a swollen rostral incisive region (*arrow*) caused by an ameloblastic carcinoma.

Compound and Complex Odontoma

An odontoma is a calcified tumor containing odontogenic epithelium and mesenchymal tissue with induction and formation of calcified enamel and dentine. These are the most differentiated dental tumors. Some other rare mixed odontogenic tumors can occur that are histologically less organized and less calcified than odontomas.[4,6]

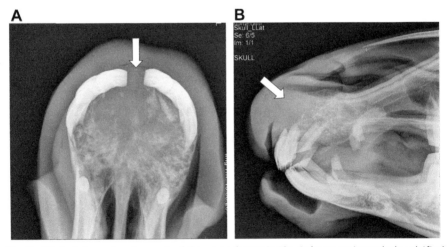

Fig. 9. (*A*) An intraoral radiograph of the pony shown in **Fig. 8** shows an irregularly calcified growth of the incisive and rostral maxillary areas, with incisor separation (*arrow*) and destruction of the adjacent cortical bone. (*B*) A lateral view showed the partially calcified growth (*arrow*) and local bone destruction. Histology of the excised mass showed an ameloblastic carcinoma. Following surgery, no regrowth occurred during a 7-year follow-up period. (Images Courtesy of Scott Dunn's Equine Clinic.)

A compound odontoma is a malformation whereby the dental tissues are in a more orderly pattern than in a complex odontoma and contain tooth-like structures (denticles).

Clinical features

These lesions more commonly affect younger horses and present as firm, painless facial swellings of the affected jaw (**Fig. 10**). If odontomas develop in the maxillary cheek teeth alveoli, they can expand into the sinuses or nasal cavity.

Diagnosis

Diagnosis is largely made by imaging that shows well-delineated, calcified growths within the jaws. If denticles are present, a compound odontoma can be definitely diagnosed (see **Fig. 10**). If denticles are absent, histology is required to differentiate a complex odontoma from other calcified dental or bone tumors.

Treatment and prognosis

Treatment is surgical excision of the well-differentiated calcified growth and any associated cyst lining and carries a good prognosis.

Cementoma (Cementoblastoma)

A cementoma is a benign, slow-growing neoplasm of cementum-producing mesenchymal cells of the periodontal tissues. Cementomas should be distinguished from the previously noted nodular hypercementosis. True cementomas are usually much larger solitary lesions, albeit at similar sites, and are not associated with periapical infections.

Diagnosis

On imaging, both cementomas and nodular hypercementosis appear as well-demarcated, usually spherical, dense radiopacities associated with the tooth apex. Histopathology of cementomas will show cemental matrix and neoplastic cementoblasts,[6] and some could be classified as hamartomas.

Treatment and prognosis

Treatment is excision of the calcified mass, exodontia of any associated tooth, and curettage of the surgical sites with a good prognosis.

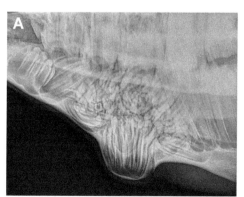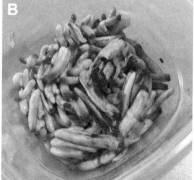

Fig. 10. (*A*) Radiographs of a 2-year-old quarter horse with a mandibular swelling of 12 months' duration show multiple denticles within the mandible. (*B*) More than 200 small, well-formed denticles were surgically resected. (Images Courtesy Jack Easley.)

BONE (OSTEOGENIC) NEOPLASIA

Osteoma
Osteosarcoma

Bone tumors, that is, *osteomas and osteosarcomas*, are rare in the horse, but many of the recorded examples occur in the head region. A juvenile ossifying fibroma is classified as a mineralized soft tissue tumor rather than a bone tumor.

Osteoma

Osteomas are slow-growing, solitary, benign bone tumors with some classified as hamartomas. Osteomas may be congenital and remain undetected if they are small or lie within the maxilla or paranasal sinuses unless they grow further or are coincidentally detected following head imaging for some other reason.

Clinical features
Equine osteomas are rounded, dense, calcified bony growths that may have a pedunculated attachment. The ventrolateral aspect of the mandible is a common site for these lesions (**Fig. 11**) that can suffer accidental trauma, including off bridles and head collars. Other osteomas may be asymptomatic, for example, within sinuses, or with growth, causing firm swellings of the facial bones.

Diagnosis
Radiography and CT imaging can usually diagnose these calcified well-demarcated lesions.

Treatment and prognosis
Surgical removal of an osteoma *may* be indicated, but some intrasinus lesions may have dense bony attachments to the reserve crowns of teeth, infraorbital canal, and facial bones and may be impossible to fully resect without damaging these structures.

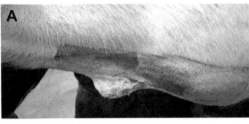
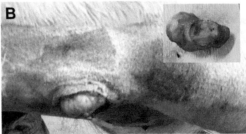

Fig. 11. (*A*) This horse had a painless hard protrusion beneath its left mandible that on radiography resembled an osteoma. (*B*) The lesion was resected under sedation and local anesthesia using a bone saw through its narrow attachment to the mandible (*inset*).

At sinusotomy, larger lesions can be sectioned using a water-cooled bone saw and osteotomes, and as much as possible can be removed in sections. The prognosis is good; even if complete removal is not achieved, recurrence is unlikely or very slow.

Osteosarcoma

Osteosarcomas are aggressive, malignant bone tumors, characterized by the presence of osteoid and immature bone created by malignant osteoblasts.[6]

Clinical features

Affected horses develop focal, possibly painful, swellings of the affected jaw (**Fig. 12**) that resemble other neoplastic or nonneoplastic jaw swellings. More aggressive lesions can cause gross bone and dental disruption, and, if in the maxilla, sinonasal and airway disruption.

Diagnosis

Imaging often shows extensive bone destruction, along with overlying periosteal new bone formation that may have the characteristic periosteal "sunburst" appearance. Histopathology of a biopsy (that can take some time to decalcify, and results may not always be definitive) is needed. Assessment of the histological degree of malignancy and of the size and site of the lesion can help decide if treatment is feasible, and if so, can help surgical planning and prognostication.[6]

Treatment and prognosis

Localized lesions in the mandible can be treated by resection of the affected section (see **Fig. 12**), but such radical resection is not possible with maxillary osteosarcomas or if a tumor has metastasized. Radiation therapy may be possible but with limited success. The prognosis is poor in most cases.

SINONASAL NEOPLASIA

Neoplasms of the sinus and nasal regions should always be considered together because these similar lesions commonly involve both of these anatomical structures. Most sinonasal tumors originate in the sinuses, especially the caudal maxillary sinus. In contrast to other species, primary nasal tumors are uncommon in horses, and some sinonasal SCC tumors originate in the oral cavity.[13] With advanced growth, it can be difficult to determine where sinonasal neoplasm originated.

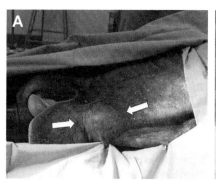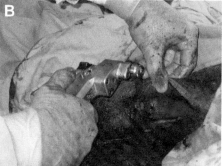

Fig. 12. (*A*) This horse presented with a swollen rostral aspect of its left mandible and a biopsy showed the presence of an osteosarcoma. (*B*) Complete resection of the affected area of the mandible was followed by mandibular stabilization with plates.

Prevalence

The prevalence of sinonasal tumors is not well documented but appears to be very low. A referral center study showed that 7.9% of 279 referred cases of sinonasal disease were due to neoplasia.[14] However, nonneoplastic space-occupying sinonasal growths, including sinus cysts, progressive ethmoid hematoma (PEH), polyps, and nasal epidermal inclusion cysts, were 3 times more prevalent, that is, comprised 23.3% of these sinonasal disease cases. A later study of 200 referred cases of paranasal sinus disease found that 5% (10/200) of sinus disease was due to neoplasia, with nonneoplastic sinus growths (mainly sinus cyst and PEH) greater than 3 times more prevalent than neoplasms.[15] A study of 300 referred cases of sinus disease that underwent head CT imaging at 3 UK referral centers showed great variation (0%, 2%, and 12%) in the prevalence of sinonasal tumors between the centers.[16]

Sinonasal Tumor Types

The clinical and pathological descriptions of 50 sinonasal neoplastic and nonneoplastic tumors recorded in the literature before 1995 included reports of individual cases and, interestingly, of endemic equine sinonasal tumors (in Sweden).[13] Non-neoplastic growths, such as maxillary (sinus) cysts, PEH, and inflammatory nasal polyps, were more commonly recorded than neoplasia.[13] The more common tumor types include SCC that, in some cases, arise in the oral cavity; adenocarcinomas; bone and odontogenic tumors; fibrosarcomas; and hemangiosarcomas. Except for some benign bone tumors, there were few records of successful treatment of equine sinonasal tumors at these times.

A study of the clinical and pathologic findings of 28 cases of equid sinonasal tumors[17] included 7 SCCs, 5 adenocarcinomas, 3 undifferentiated carcinomas, 2 adenomas, 5 fibro-osseous (ossifying fibroma) and bone tumors, and single cases of ameloblastoma, fibroma, fibrosarcoma, undifferentiated sarcoma, melanoma, and lymphosarcoma. The median ages of animals affected with epithelial and fibro-osseous/bone tumors were 14 and 4 years, respectively.

The maxillary area was the most common site of tumor origin, and only 3 of 28 cases were definitively identified as originating in the nasal cavity, and 2 (SCCs) originated in the oral cavity. Unilateral purulent or mucopurulent nasal discharge (81% of cases) and gross facial swellings (82% of cases) were the most common presenting signs, with epistaxis recorded in just 23% of cases. Radiography and endoscopy were the most useful ancillary diagnostic techniques.[17] CT, which provides more information on sinonasal tumor size, features of malignancy, and important prognostic indicators,[8] was unavailable at that time.

Fourteen of 15 carcinomas, but only 2 of the 13 remaining tumors, spread to other sites in the head. Only 3 of 23 cases of sinonasal tumors had lymph node metastases recorded, and none had distant metastases. In the long term, surgical treatment with 7 malignant tumors was unsuccessful (6 months median survival postoperatively) but was successful with 4 out of 5 benign tumors (no regrowth at a median of 4 years postoperatively).[17]

Cissell and colleagues[8] described the CT appearance of 15 equine sinonasal tumors, including 5 neuroendocrine tumors/neuroblastomas, 2 undifferentiated carcinomas, 2 myxosarcomas, and one each of nasal adenocarcinoma, hemangiosarcoma, chondroblastic osteosarcoma, anaplastic sarcoma, myxoma, and ossifying fibroma. These types of tumors differed from the more commonly reported tumors of this region.

Nonneoplastic Sinonasal Growths

As noted, non-neoplastic sinonasal growths, mainly PEH and sinus cysts, are about 3 times more common than true sinonasal neoplasms.

Progressive Ethmoid Hematoma

PEHs are best pathologically described as hemorrhagic polyps, and their stroma has the histological appearance of a recurring hematoma. PEH lesions are the most common cause of chronic, low-grade unilateral epistaxis in horses. They usually affect adults and most commonly develop on the rostral aspect of the nasal ethmoturbinates and appear as multicolored yellow/green or red/blue smooth, rounded masses protruding rostrally into the nasal cavity (**Fig. 13**). Less commonly, they grow laterally or dorsally from the lateral aspect of the ethmoid mass into the caudal maxillary and conchofrontal, or less commonly, into the sphenopalatine sinuses.

Mucopurulent as well as hemorrhagic nasal discharge can occur. Airflow obstruction, facial swelling, and neurological signs (because of sphenopalatine sinus involvement) are rare. Diagnosis is readily made by nasal endoscopy (see **Fig. 13**) or sinoscopy by visualizing the very characteristic lesions. CT shows a well-circumscribed mass with mineralization of the capsule surrounding mixed soft tissue densities with hyperattenuating reticular patterns. Treatment can be by transendoscopic infiltration of their attachment sites with cytotoxic materials, such as formalin, or by surgical excision.

Sinus Cysts

Sinus cysts are fluid-filled cysts that usually develop in the maxillary and occasionally in the frontal sinuses and can occur in all age groups. Very marked unilateral facial swelling, epiphora, and nasal airflow obstruction are the main clinical features, and these greatly resemble the signs of sinonasal neoplasia (**Fig. 14**). Obstruction to normal sinus mucous flow can cause secondary sinus infection, and thus mucopurulent nasal discharge can later occur. Diagnosis can be confirmed by radiography or more readily by aspiration of straw-colored fluid after inserting a 16-gauge

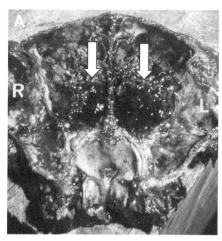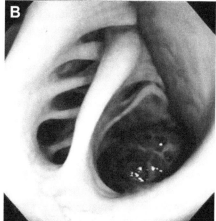

Fig. 13. (*A*) Postmortem image of a transverse section of a horse's head shows bilateral PEH lesions in the ethmoid masses (*arrows*). (*B*) This nasal endoscopic image shows a small PEH lesion lying between the nasal ethmoturbinates.

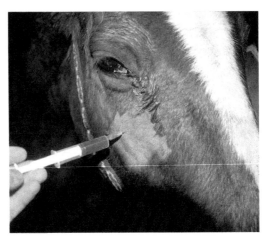

Fig. 14. A young horse is having aspiration of its swollen, right maxillary area using a needle inserted through softened bone. Clear, pale-yellow fluid is being readily aspirated, confirming the presence of a sinus cyst.

hypodermic needle into the thinned bone overlying the facial swelling. As always, CT is the optimal imaging modality for the complicated 3-dimensional structure of the sinonasal region. Cyst excision by maxillary or nasofrontal osteotomy or by sinoscopy for smaller lesions gives excellent results.[18]

SINONASAL NEOPLASIA
Introduction

Equine nasal and sinus tumors are best considered together, as they are the same types of tumors, that is, usually highly malignant epithelial neoplasms, and with time, they often involve both the nasal and the sinus compartments. The different types of sinonasal neoplasms cause similar signs as they expand within the sinonasal region. An exception are SCC tumors that can initially develop in the oral cavity where they can readily be visualized and biopsied (**Fig. 15**). Oral examination (also for detection of dental disease) should be an essential part of the clinical examination of every horse with sinonasal disease.

Clinical Signs

The clinical signs initially reflect local expansive pressure changes within the sinuses or nasal cavity, along with inflammation and secondary infection of tissues damaged by the tumor. Tumor expansion can cause facial swelling. Obstruction of normal sinonasal mucous drainage along with secondary infection of invaded tissue leads to sinus empyema. This causes a malodorous unilateral mucopurulent/purulent nasal discharge, which rarely may progress to an intermittent bilateral discharge if one nasal cavity becomes obstructed. Nasal airflow obstruction also occurs with bilateral nasal involvement. Epistaxis is uncommon, unlike sinonasal neoplasia in other species. Unilateral submandibular lymph node enlargement is invariably present, mainly because of sinonasal infection and inflammation, rather than because of metastases. Many clinical signs are similar to those of nonneoplastic sinonasal growths, such as sinus cysts.

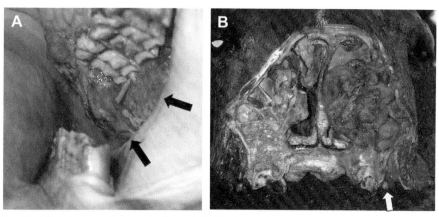

Fig. 15. (*A*) An intraoral view of a large left-sided maxillary area SCC (*arrows*). (*B*) This postmortem image of an equine head shows the left-sided sinus compartments and nasal cavity to have extensive neoplasia (SCC) that originated in the oral cavity (*arrow*).

Diagnosis

Imaging of the affected region, especially by CT if available,[6,8] is of greatest value in diagnosis and prognostication. Nasal endoscopy may show exudate draining from the sinonasal ostium or evidence of nasal airway compression, and rarely, an intranasal mass. Biopsy using transendoscopic forceps *may* obtain a suitable sample of

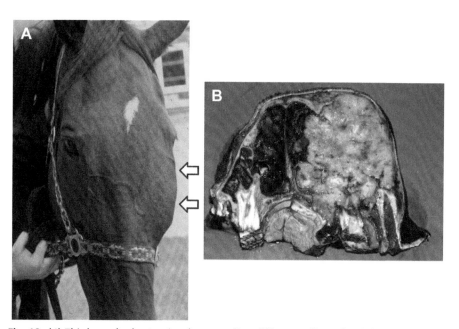

Fig. 16. (*A*) This horse had extensive, longstanding diffuse swelling of its left maxillary and frontal areas (*arrows*), along with nasal airflow obstruction. (*B*) Postmortem examination shows a very extensive, left-sided firm sinonasal growth. Although it was a benign ossifying fibroma, it was so extensive that surgery was not possible.

a nasal mass for histology. Sinoscopy under standing sedation allows a suitable biopsy of an intrasinus mass to be obtained.

Treatment and Prognosis

Most equine soft tissue sinonasal tumors cannot be successfully surgically treated owing to extensive invasion by the time they are diagnosed, and thus, euthanasia is often indicated.[4,6,15,16] Some benign fibro-osseous (ossifying fibromas) lesions that in theory should be capable of excision are so extensive by the time of diagnosis that they are also impossible to treat (**Fig. 16**), but smaller benign lesions can be successfully resected.[16] Radiotherapy and intralesional cytotoxic therapy can be considered for these tumors, as discussed elsewhere in this issue.

DISCLOSURE

The author has nothing to disclose.

REFERENCES

1. Pascoe RR, Summers PM. Clinical survey of tumors and tumorlike lesions in horses in southeast Queensland. Equine Vet J 1981;13:2358.
2. Cotchin E. A general survey of tumors in the horse. Equine Vet J 1977;9:16–21.
3. Pirie RS, Dixon PM. Mandibular tumors in the horse: a review of the literature and 7 case reports. Equine Vet Educ 1993;5:287–94.
4. Knottenbelt DC, Snalune K, Kane JP. In: Knottenbelt DC, Snalune K, Kane JP, editors. Clinical equine oncology. 1st edition. Edinburgh: Elsevier Health Sciences; 2015. p. pp429–511.
5. Morgan RE, Fiske-Jackson AR, Hellige M, et al. Equine odontogenic tumors: Clinical presentation, CT findings, and outcome in 11 horses. Vet Radiol Ultrasound 2019;60:502–12.
6. Bienert-Zeit A, Rawlinson J, Bell C. Oral, nasal and sinus masses. In: Easley Jack, editor. Padraic Dixon and Nicole du Toit Equine Dentistry and Maxillofacial Surgery. 1st edition; 2022. p. 236–73. Chapter 14.
7. Dixon PM, Loh N, Barakzai SZ. Swellings of the angle of the mandible in 32 horses (1997–2011). Vet J 2014;199:97–102.
8. Cissell DD, Wisner DR, Textor J, et al. Computed tomographic appearance of equine sinonasal neoplasia. Vet Radiol Ultrasound 2012;53:245–51.
9. Horbal A, Dixon PM. Gingival Fibrosarcoma in a Horse. J Vet Dent 2016;33: 243–8.
10. Haion O, Tatz A, Brenner O, et al. Rostral mandibulectomy as a treatment for comminuted pars incisiva fractures and fibro-osseous lesions: A retrospective study including six cases. Equine Vet Educ 2023;35:e706–12.
11. Reardon RJM, Dixon PM, Kane-Smyth J, et al. Combined surgical and radiotherapy treatment of a mandibular ameloblastic carcinoma in a pony. Equine Ve Educ 2017;29:641–6.
12. Brounts SH, Hawkins JF, Lescun TB, et al. Surgical management of compound odontoma in two horses. J Am Vet Med Assoc 2004;225:1423–7.
13. Head KW, Dixon PM. Equine nasal and paranasal sinus tumors. Part 1: review of the literature and tumour classification. Vet J 1999;157:261–78.
14. Tremaine WH, Dixon PM. A long-term study of 277 cases of equine sinonasal disease. Part 1: details of horses, historical, clinical and ancillary diagnostic findings. Equine Vet J 2001;33:274–82.

15. Dixon PM, Parkin TD, Collins N, et al. Equine paranasal sinus disease - a long-term study of 200 cases (1997-2009): ancillary diagnostic findings and involvement of the various sinus compartments. Equine Vet J 2012;44:267–71.
16. Dixon PM, Barnett TP, Morgan RE, et al. Computed tomographic assessment of individual paranasal sinus compartment and nasal conchal bulla involvement in 300 cases of equine sinonasal disease. Frontiers Vet Sci 2020;7:580356.
17. Dixon PM, Head KW. Equine Nasal and Paranasal Sinus Tumors: Part 2: A Contribution of 28 Case Reports. Vet J 1999;157:279–94.
18. Woodford N, Lane J. Long-term retrospective study of 52 horses with sinonasal cysts. Equine Vet J 2006;38:198–202.

Equine Gastrointestinal Neoplasia

Ina Mersich, Mag med vet, Pamela A. Wilkins, DVM, MS, PhD*

KEYWORDS

- Esophageal • Gastric • Intestinal • Pancreatic • Hepatic • Splenic • Tumor
- Cancer

KEY POINTS

- Gastrointestinal neoplasia is uncommon in horses.
- Clinical signs can be vague and advanced testing, including biopsy, exploratory surgery, and/or advanced imaging may be required for diagnosis.
- Prognosis varies by location, organ involved, and is frequently poor to grave.

INTRODUCTION

Gastrointestinal neoplasia is rare in equine patients.[1] Most commonly found tumors of the equine gastrointestinal tract are alimentary lymphoma, intestinal adenocarcinoma, intestinal leiomyoma, and leiomyosarcoma; and squamous cell carcinoma (SCC)—when involving the esophagus or stomach.[2,3] Clinical signs are variable and often nonspecific, but frequently include weight loss, inappetence, lethargy, colic, increased vital signs, and diarrhea.[4–11] Clinicopathological abnormalities are generally not tumor-specific and commonly consist of anemia, hypoproteinemia, hyperglobulinemia, hypoalbuminemia, leukogram abnormalities, hyperfibrinogenemia, hyperbilirubinemia, electrolyte derangements, increased liver enzymes, and hyperphosphatemia[10,12–15] Tumor-specific findings are listed with each type in the following sections. Helpful diagnostic tools are transabdominal ultrasonography, rectal examination, abdominocentesis, histopathology, immunohistochemistry, and laparotomy/necropsy[4–7,12] Frequently observed ultrasonographic changes encompass enlarged mesenteric lymph nodes, intestinal thickening or distension, peritoneal effusion and masses within abdominal organs, soft tissue, mesentery, and peritoneum.[5,12,16–19]

Rectal examination may reveal mesenteric nodules or thickening, peritoneal effusion, intra-abdominal masses, enlarged mesenteric lymph nodes and intestinal

Department of Veterinary Clinical Medicine, University of Illinois, 1008 West Hazelwood Drive, Urbana, IL 61802, USA
* Coresponding author.
E-mail address: pawilkin@illinois.edu

Vet Clin Equine 40 (2024) 475–485
https://doi.org/10.1016/j.cveq.2024.07.011
0749-0739/24/© 2024 Elsevier Inc. All rights reserved, including those for text and data mining, AI training, and similar technologies.

thickening or distension.[5–8,12,20,21] Abdominal fluid analysis is largely nonspecific, but may show neoplastic effusion, increased total cell count and protein, mitotic figures or non-septic exudate.[5,12] Histopathology often shows neoplastic cells, high mitotic indices, necrosis, or hemorrhage.[22] Immunohistochemistry can be used to characterize tumor and tissue types.[4] Treatment options are generally limited and mentioned when reported for a specific tumor type. Prognosis is generally reported as poor, except for non-metastasizing resectable tumors.[4,6,23,24]

ESOPHAGUS

SCC, leiomyoma, and melanoma have been reported to affect the equine esophagus.[22,25] Tumor-specific clinical signs are esophageal obstruction, nasal discharge, dysphagia, and hemoptyalism.[4,22] Diagnosis is facilitated by esophagoscopy, native/contrast radiography, or computed tomography.[22,25,26]

SCC arises from epithelial cells, specifically keratinocytes, and occurs rarely in horses.[4] Esophagoscopy may reveal esophageal narrowing, masses, wall irregularities, ulcerations, or hyperemia.[22] Tissue staining during endoscopy with Lugol's iodine and toluidine blue may aid diagnosis.[27] Native and contrast radiography are helpful and mucosal irregularities, stricture, and dilation have been reported. At necropsy, mucosal thickening, ulceration, and papilliform/verrucous lesions can be seen.[22]

Leiomyomas are benign tumors, derived from smooth muscle cells with slow growth tendency and rare in horses. Inciting causes are unknown, but chronic trauma (epiglottic entrapment) or toxin ingestion are possible. Clinical signs include feed-containing nasal discharge (choke) and, rarely, respiratory signs. Endoscopy, radiography, and histopathology are useful diagnostic tools. Masses tend to be well demarcated and involve muscular layers.[28]

Primary esophageal melanoma has been reported once. Tumor-related clinical signs were not reported and the necropsy finding was considered incidental. Congenital neoplasia was considered likely versus placental transmission of metastatic melanoma. Esophageal thickening and black appearance of a well-demarcated mass were found.[25]

STOMACH

Gastric tumors are relatively uncommon, accounting for less than 2% of equine neoplasia, with SCC and lymphoma the most common diagnoses. Others include adenocarcinoma, leiomyosarcoma, stromal tumors, and papillomas. Presentation age varies, with middle-aged to older horses being more frequently affected and duration ranging from weeks to years. Hypersalivation, halitosis, dysphagia, bruxism, or edema may be encountered.[2,5,29,30]

SCC is the most common gastric neoplasia reported in horses and originates from the squamous mucosa.[5] Recently *Equus caballus papillomavirus-2* has been identified in a subset of primary gastric SCC and metastasis.[31] Clinically, malodorous reflux has been reported aside from nonspecific findings.[20] Clinicopathological alterations mostly reflect chronic inflammation and/or hemorrhage.[5,12,13,16] Metastasis is common (occurrence up to 68%), involving multiple intra-abdominal organs (omentum, peritoneal cavity, lymph nodes, spleen, liver, pleural cavity, pericardium, and thymus). Carcinomatosis, hematogenous/lymphatic metastasis, and local invasion have been reported with metastasis.[5,12,13,32,33] Pleural effusion and hypertrophic osteopathy have been reported.[13,33] During gastroscopy, masses, hyperemia, stenosis, mucosal erosions, and proliferation may be found. In up to 57% of cases abdominocentesis may show neoplastic effusion and non-nucleated keratinized cells. Transabdominal ultrasonography might reveal gastric masses, distension, wall thickening, and irregularity. Biopsies are diagnostically useful and can be obtained endoscopy-guided, transcutaneous ultrasound-guided, transcutaneous (accessible organ metastasis) or during exploratory laparotomy. Necropsy and histopathology findings are diagnostic.[5,12,20,32] Treatment is generally discouraged due to grave prognosis (71% subjected to euthanasia) and welfare concerns, but may be attempted palliatively. Piroxicam is used with canine oral SCC, reducing prostaglandin E synthesis, and has been suggested for treatment of equine gastric SCC although successful cases are not reported to date. Dexamethasone is another palliative option.[4,12,34]

Leiomyoma is a benign tumor, and leiomyosarcoma a malignant tumor of gastric smooth muscle. Metastasis is not reported with leiomyoma, leiomyosarcoma is locally invasive and slowly metastasizing. Clinically recurrent colic is most commonly reported. Diagnosis can be challenging, gastroscopy may not reveal abnormalities, but exploratory laparotomy can aid diagnosis. Masses with muscularis origin possibly extending to mucosa, which may be irregular and necrotic, are possible necropsy findings. Prognosis is poor, although both tumors progress slowly.[4,5,35]

Gastric adenocarcinoma emerges from the glandular crypt epithelium. Few reports about metastasis exist. Colic is most commonly reported; however, hepatic encephalopathy due to secondary portal vein metastasis and thrombosis was present in one case.[4,5,36] Small masses of gastric serosa and greater curvature (local extension) have been reported.[5,29] Cases present late in the disease process, prognosis is therefore poor.[4]

Gastric lymphoma arises from the gastric submucosa. Peripheral lymph node biopsy and subsequent histopathology, if lymph node involvement is present, can aid diagnosis.[5]

Gastric stromal tumor has been associated with ataxia, collapse, muscle wasting, and hypoglycemia among nonspecific signs in one case. A large mass between stomach, liver, and colon with stalky attachment to the stomach was found.[37]

INTESTINE

Intestinal tumors include lymphoma, adenocarcinoma, leiomyosarcoma, leiomyoma, stromal tumors, and hemangioma. Aside from common signs associated with neoplasia, patchy sweating, lymphadenopathy, ventral edema, ascites, respiratory distress, diarrhea, and melena have been described.[6–8,38]

Lymphoma is the most common equine neoplasm.[4] Within the alimentary form, the small intestine is most commonly affected, with T-cell lymphomas being most frequent.[39] Lymphoma types include

T-cell lymphoma (enteropathy-associated T-cell lymphoma type I and II, peripheral T-cell lymphoma).
B-cell lymphoma (diffuse large B-cell lymphoma, T-cell–rich large B-cell lymphoma).[40]
Large granular lymphoma (uncommon).
Diffuse large-cell lymphoma[41]

Intestinal lymphoma likely emerges from mucosal lymphoid tissue.[4] Secondary complications include intra-abdominal metastasis, lymphomatosis, multifocal pseudodiverticula, transcolonic fistulas, or strangulating lesions. Lymphoid-rich organs like spleen, bone marrow, and pharynx are predisposed for metasasis.[7,42–45]

Peritoneal lymphomatosis, although rare, has been reported in horses.[46] Cytology of lymph node aspirate or biopsy is diagnostically helpful and small intestinal malabsorption was reported in several cases.[4,47] Peritoneal lymphocytosis has been reported and rectal biopsy may be diagnostic.[7,17,18,44] Intestinal thickening, mesenteric lymph node enlargement, nodules or plaques, hyperplastic Peyer's patches, mucosal erosion/ulceration, and intestinal diverticula may be encountered during laparotomy/necropsy.[7,17,39,41,48] The intestine may contain short/absent villi, leukocytes within crypts and mucosal/submucosal lymphoid infiltration. Mesenteric lymph nodes can show extensive lymphoid tissue and necrotic–hemorrhagic lymphadenitis.[17,49] The diagnostic use of serum thymidine kinase in equine lymphoma is controversial, with one study showing promising results[32] and another one revealing no association.[50] EHV-5 has been identified in one case of intestinal lymphoma and several with other affected organs/tissues.[17,45] Treatment may be attempted, even though mostly palliative.[4] Alimentary and multicentric lymphoma showed the lowest success rate.[51] Chemotherapeutic drugs have been suggested, although data for the treatment and outcome are lacking.[4] Doxorubicin is an anti-tumor antibiotic that has cytotoxic properties inhibiting DNA and RNA synthesis. It has been used successfully in horses with lymphoma, but reports did not specify lymphoma type.[4,52,53] Other options include cyclophosphamide, vincristine, L-asparaginase, lomustine, cytosine arabinoside, and corticosteroids. Surgical resection of solitary masses may be attempted. With large intestinal involvement, colon resection has been reported in two cases. Outcome and long-term survival are poor due to late presentation.[4,54]

Intestinal adenocarcinoma is the second most common intestinal neoplasia, arising from the glandular crypt epithelium of the intestine, and reports differ between predispositions for large or small intestine. It has been reported mostly in older horses and Arabian breeds.[3,4,6] Intestinal adenocarcinoma may metastasize into the thorax, spleen, liver, diaphragm, peritoneum, and skeleton.[55,56] Hematochezia and melena was noted in several cases.[38] Anemia and osseous metaplasia are commonly found and concurrent enteric clostridiosis was reported once.[8,19,21,57,58] Abdominal fluid may contain neoplastic cells in acinar patterns and intra-abdominal inflammation.[55] Colonic thickening and irregularity with heterogenic areas may be found ultrasonographically.[58] Necropsy may reveal pleural effusion, adhesions, and obstruction caused by intestinal masses and organ rupture due to neoplastic invasion.[8,55,59] Multiple abdominal organs may be affected. Successful surgical tumor excision has been reported and may prolong life expectancy.[1,3,4,58,60] Prognosis depends on disease progression.

Intestinal leiomyoma/leiomyosarcoma arise from intestinal smooth muscle layers and have been reported to involve the jejunum, duodenum, large and small colon, and cecum. They present as smooth, encapsulated, and solitary masses[3,23,61–63] and make up around 15% of intestinal neoplasms.[6] Laparotomy/necropsy may show masses causing volvulus, adhesions, or obstruction by annular intestinal thickening and concurrent polyps.[23,61–64] Surgical excision of jejunal and colonic leiomyosarcoma and small colon leiomyoma have been reported.[6,23,65]

Gastrointestinal stromal tumors (GIST) are mesenchymal tumors composed of nondifferentiated mesenchymal cells, with mature myogenic, myofibroblastic or neural components primarily seen in older horses. They have been identified in the ileum, jejunum, cecum, and large colon, and make up around 15% of equine intestinal tumors. GIST may be underrepresented due to difficulty differentiating them from smooth muscle tumors. In a report of 11 affected horses, no metastasis were observed.[6,24] Masses may appear heterogenic and solid on ultrasound. Necropsy findings include intramural/subserosal masses, possibly pedunculated or cystic, and a rather invasive nature. Surgical resection of a mass with associated strangulated small intestine has been reported.[24,65–67]

Intestinal nerve sheath tumors include neurofibroma, schwannoma, perineurioma, nerve sheath myxoma, and other peripheral nerve tumors.[4] In the equine gastrointestinal tract, they have been reported in the colon and the small intestine. Epiploic foramen entrapment, due to abnormal gastrointestinal motility associated with several nerve sheath tumors and hyperplastic enteric plexuses have been reported.[68]

Ganglioneuroma tumors arise from the sympathetic nervous system.[69] One case report found a jejunal mass, causing intestinal strangulation. The mass was successfully removed and composed of ganglion cells.[70]

Metastatic melanoma may involve several intra-abdominal organs including the spleen, liver, mesentery, omentum, and intestinal serosa, and present as round/oval masses with black pigment. Histopathology shows neoplastic melanocytes.[71]

MESENTERY AND PERITONEUM

Lipomatosis differs from discrete lipomas, resulting in tissue infiltrates and expansion.[72] The terms infiltrative lipoma and lipomatosis are used interchangeably. Lipomatosis, although benign, can cause tissue infiltration and intestinal obstruction/compromise. Infiltrative lesions of intestinal muscle and nervous tissue can cause weakening and intestinal wall herniation, leading to impactions and intestinal rupture.[73] Lipomatosis can affect both the mesentery and intestines. Ultrasonography may reveal multilobulation, tissue splitting or stacked masses with fat-like echogenicity.[72,74–76] Laparotomy/necropsy may show abundant retroperitoneal fat, discrete lipomas, fat accumulation or masses within intestines or mesentery, obstruction, and intestinal diverticula caused by fat infiltration/accumulation.[73–75]

Mesotheliomas are malignant tumors originating from mesothelial cells (peritoneal, pleural, pericardial, or scrotal). In the abdomen they commonly arise from the greater omentum.[4] Epithelioid, biphasic, and sarcomatoid types are known. Lipid-rich mesothelioma is a morphologic variant of the epithelioid form and has been reported in one horse. Tumor-lysis syndrome and paraneoplastic hypoglycemia were diagnosed in one horse, showing metabolic abnormalities and renal failure. Mesotheliomas tend to exfoliate and severe peritoneal effusion is a key clinical finding, making abdominocentesis diagnostically valuable. Clinical signs frequently include ascites and abdominal distension. Ultrasonographically cauliflower-shaped masses adjacent to the abdominal wall and mesenteric and splenic masses have been observed. Multilobular peritoneal, hepatic or splenic masses, omental thickening, and mesenteric lymph node involvement may be found.[14,77–81]

PANCREAS

Pancreatic adenocarcinoma is commonly associated with liver dysfunction/liver enzyme increase, likely related to the anatomic association between liver and pancreas. Hyperammonemia has also been reported. Metastatic lesions include pleural effusion, peritoneal and retroperitoneal organs, lymph nodes, aorta, and adrenal glands. Necropsy findings incorporate pancreatic or abdominal masses and metastatic lesions. The non-neoplastic pancreas may appear fibrotic.[9,82]

Malignant glucagonoma has been reported in one horse presented for chronic weight loss, tachycardia, tachypnea, and muscle wasting. Clinicopathological abnormalities included increased GGT, hyperglycemia and glucosuria aside from nonspecific changes. No pancreatic mass was found despite the strong suspicion.[83]

LIVER

Hepatoblastoma, hamartoma, hepatocellular carcinoma, and cholangiocarcinoma have been reported in horses. Primary hepatic neoplasia has been diagnosed in young horses and fetuses. Clinical signs and laboratory abnormalities commonly indicate liver disease including polycythemia, increased liver enzymes, hyperbilirubinemia, increased bile acids, and hyperammonemia. Abdominal ultrasonography may reveal hepatomegaly, rounded liver edges, heterogeneous parenchyma and loss of structure and gastric metastasis has been reported.[15,20,84–89]

Hepatoblastoma is an embryonal tumor likely derived from hepatocyte precursors.[50] Paraneoplastic manifestations including polycythemia and stress fractures have been observed. Liver masses, hepatomegaly, ascites, organ congestion, and portal vein thrombosis may be seen. Metastasis can include lymph nodes, skin, brain, meninges, bones, peritoneal and visceral surfaces of peritoneal organs, and lungs. Treatment is mainly symptomatic. Reported cases either died, were euthanized, or were stillborn feti. Treatment for erythrocytosis has been attempted with intravenous fluid therapy, phlebotomy, and blood removal with minimal improvement.[15,84–86,90–92]

Hepatocellular carcinoma is of hepatocellular origin.[4] On necropsy, ascites, liver masses, hepatomegaly, and metastasis to the hepatic vein, diaphragm, omentum, serosal surfaces of spleen and abdominal wall, lung, kidney, and lymph nodes have been reported.[84,87]

Cholangiocarcinoma is a malignant tumor arising from intrahepatic biliary epithelial cells.[4] Combinations of cholangiocarcinoma with SCC of the stomach and hepatocellular carcinoma have been reported.[20,93] Affected horses are aged rather than young.[89] Necropsy findings include nodular liver masses, hepatomegaly, and enlarged abdominal lymph nodes. Metastasis may affect the peritoneum, omental, and serosal surfaces of diaphragm, spleen, and stomach.[20,89]

Biliary adenofibroma is a benign tumor originating from the biliary epithelium, with only one case reported to date. Necropsy revealed a solid and oval hepatic tumor including several small cysts.[94]

Hepatic hamartoma is a benign tumor reported in equine feti as a mixed or mesenchymal type. Necropsy showed hepatomegaly; firm, tan, and reticular liver appearance or circumscribed masses. Observed histopathological lesions were consistent with mesenchymal hamartoma, some features resembling congenital hepatic fibrosis.[95,96]

SPLEEN

Reported primary tumors are lymphoma and hemangiosarcoma. Due to abundant blood supply and organ functions, splenic metastasis is common. Frequently metastasizing tumors are melanoma, hemangiosarcoma, and lymphoma.[4,69]

Splenic lymphoma with pseudohyperparathyroidism due to paraneoplastic syndrome leading to polyuria and polydypsia has been reported. Splenomegaly and splenic displacement may be palpated rectally. Ultrasonography might show hyperechoic nodules containing anechoic areas, capsule irregularities, and heterogenic masses within the spleen.[10,11]

Splenic hemangiosarcoma derives from the vascular system and may appear as a primary splenic tumor or metastasis. Associated clinical and clinicopathological abnormalities include anemia, leukocytosis, thrombocytopenia, and changes associated with abdominal distension/hemorrhage. Abdominocentesis may reveal hemoabdomen or neoplastic effusion. Splenic biopsy or fine needle aspirate is most diagnostic. Reported treatment has been supportive and unsuccessful. Splenectomy is theoretically feasible, but has not been reported.[4,69]

CLINICS CARE POINTS

- Equine gastrointestinal neoplasia is an uncommon finding and often carries a grave prognosis due to presentation late in the disease process.
- Common clinical findings are often unspecific and include weight loss, inappetence, colic and lethargy.
- Clinicopathological findings can be unspecific and commonly include anemia, hypoproteinemia, hyperglobulinemia and hypoalbuminemia.
- Useful diagnostic aids are ultrasonography, endoscopy, histopathology and exploratory laparotomy.
- Treatment options are scarce and often unsuccessful.

DISCLOSURE

No conflicts of interest to declare.

REFERENCES

1. East LM, Savage CJ. Abdominal Neoplasia. Vet Clin N Am 1998;3:475–93.
2. Sundberg JP, Burnstein T, Page EH, et al. Neoplasms of Equidae. J Am Vet Med Assoc 1977;2:150–2.
3. Taylor SD, Pusterla N, Vaughan B, et al. Intestinal Neoplasia in Horses. J Vet Intern Med 2006;6:1429–36.
4. Derek C, Knottenbelt J, Patterson-Kane C, et al. Clinical equine oncology. Edinburgh: Elsevier; 2015. p. 679.
5. Taylor SD, Haldorson GJ, Vaughan B, et al. Gastric Neoplasia in Horses. J Vet Intern Med 2009;23(5):1097–102.
6. Spanton JA, Smith LJ, Sherlock CE, et al. Intestinal neoplasia: A review of 34 cases. Equine Vet Educ 2020;3:155–65.
7. Mair TS, Hillyer MH. Clinical features of lymphosarcoma in the horse: 77 cases. Equine Vet Educ 1992;3:108–13.
8. Völker I, Puschmann T, Michutta J, et al. Intestinal adenocarcinoma in ponies: Clinical and pathological findings. Equine Vet Educ 2018;12:630–4.
9. Church S, West HJ, Baker JR. Two cases of pancreatic adenocarcinoma in horses. Equine Vet J 1987;1:77–9.
10. Marr C. Clinical, ultrasonographic and pathological findings in a horse with splenic lymphosarcoma and pseudohyperparathyroidism. Equine Vet J 1989;3:221–6.
11. Hananeh W. Primary splenic diffuse large B-cell lymphoma with multinucleated giant cells in a horse. Vet Med 2021;2:76–9.
12. Rocafort Ferrer G, Nolf M, Belluco S, et al. Gastric squamous cell carcinoma in the horse: Seven cases (2009–2019). Equine Vet Educ 2021;10:357–64.
13. McKenzie E, Mills J, Bolton J. Gastric squamous cell carcinoma in three horses. Aust Vet J 1997;7:480–3.
14. LaCarrubba AM, Johnson PJ, Whitney MS, et al. Hypoglycemia and Tumor Lysis Syndrome Associated with Peritoneal Mesothelioma in a Horse. J Vet Intern Med 2006;4:1018–22.
15. Lennox TJ, Wilson JH, Hayden DW, et al. Hepatoblastoma with erythrocytosis in a young female horse. J Am Vet Med Assoc 2000;5:718–21.

16. Tennant B, Keirn DR, White KK, et al. Six cases of squamous cell carcinoma of the stomach of the horse. Equine Vet J 1982;3:238–43.
17. Miglio A, Morelli C, Gialletti R, et al. Clinical and immunophenotypic findings in 4 forms of equine lymphoma. Canadian Vet J 2019;1:33–40.
18. Sherlock C, Dawson L, Mair T. Ultrasound as a diagnostic tool in the investigation of a pony with intestinal lymphoma. Equine Vet Educ 2017;2:78–81.
19. Maalouf R, Alonso-Sousa S, Graham R. Colonic adenocarcinoma resulting in recurrent colic and hematochezia in an Arabian stallion. Vlaams Diergeneeskd Tijdschr 2020;3:138–43.
20. Pizzigatti D, Batista FA, Martins CF, et al. Cholangiocarcinoma and Squamous Cell Carcinoma of the Stratified Epithelial Portion of the Stomach in a Horse: A Case Report. J Equine Vet Sci 2011;31(1):3–7.
21. Harvey-Micay J. Intestinal adenocarcinoma causing recurrent colic in the horse. Can Vet J 1999;10:729–30.
22. Roberts MC. Squamous cell carcinoma of the lower cervical esophagus in a pony. Equine Vet J 1979;3:199–201.
23. Haven ML, Rottman JB, Bowman KF. Leiomyoma of the Small Colon in a Horse. Vet Surg 1991;5:320–2.
24. Del Piero F, Summers BA, Cummings JF, et al. Gastrointestinal Stromal Tumors in Equids. Vet Pathol 2001;6:689–97.
25. Caston SS, Fales-Williams A. Primary malignant melanoma in the oesophagus of a foal. Equine Vet Educ 2010;8:387–90.
26. Brazil TJ. Recurrent oesophageal obstruction caused by gastrooesophageal squamous carcinoma: A diagnostic challenge for the clinician? Equine Vet Educ 2008;12:633–4.
27. Green EM. Esophageal obstruction. In: Robinson NE, editor. Current therapy in equine medicine. 3rd edn. Philadelphia: W.B. Saunders; 1992. p. 175–84.
28. Faulkner J, Vlaminck L, Geerinck L, et al. Leiomyoma of the proximal cervical oesophagus in a horse. Equine Vet Educ 2022;3:154–9.
29. Patton KM, Peek SF, Valentine BA. Gastric Adenocarcinoma in a Horse with Portal Vein Metastasis and Thrombosis: A Novel Cause of Hepatic Encephalopathy. Vet Pathol 2006;4:565–9.
30. Marley LK, Repenning P, Frank CB, et al. Transendoscopic Electrosurgery for Partial Removal of a Gastric Adenomatous Polyp in a Horse. J Vet Intern Med 2016;4: 1351–5.
31. Alloway E, Linder K, May S, et al. A subset of equine gastric squamous cell carcinomas is associated with Equus caballus papillomavirus-2. Vet Pathol 2020;3: 427–31.
32. Straticò P, Razzuoli E, Hattab J, et al. Equine Gastric Squamous Cell Carcinoma in a Friesian Stallion. J Equine Vet Sci 2022;117:104087.
33. Schleining JA, Voss ED. Hypertrophic osteopathy secondary to gastric squamous cell carcinoma in a horse. Equine Vet Educ 2010;6:304–7.
34. Elce YA, Orsini JA, Blikslager AT. Expression of cyclooxygenase-1 and -2 in naturally occurring squamous cell carcinomas in horses. Am J Vet Res 2007;1:76–80.
35. Boy MG, Heyer G, Hamir AN. Gastric leiomyosarcoma in a horse. J Am Vet Med Assoc 1992;9:1363–4.
36. Cotchin E. A General Survey of Tumours in the Horse. Equine Vet J 1977;1:16–21.
37. Haga HA, Ytrehus B, Rudshaug IJ, et al. Gastrointestinal stromal tumour and hypoglycemia in a Fjord pony: Case report. Acta veterinaria scandinavia 2009; 1:1–5.
38. Metcalfe A, Craig LE. Intestinal hemangiomas in 8 horses. Vet Pathol 2022;2:1–4.

39. Bacci B, Stent AW, Walmsley EA. Equine Intestinal Lymphoma: Clinical-Pathological Features, Immunophenotype, and Survival. Vet Pathol 2020;3: 369–76.

40. Durham AC, Pillitteri CA, Myint MS, et al. Two Hundred Three Cases of Equine Lymphoma Classified According to the World Health Organization (WHO) Classification Criteria. Vet Pathol 2013;1:86–93.

41. Sheats MK, Wetter AJNJV, Snyder LA, et al. Disseminated large granular lymphoma in a horse. Equine Vet Educ 2008;9:459–63.

42. Matsuda K, Shimada T, Kawamura Y, et al. Jejunal Intussusception Associated with Lymphoma in a Horse. J Vet Med Sci 2013;9:1253–6.

43. Perry LR, Butler AJ, John E, et al. Lymphomatosis as a Cause of Abdominal Pain and Distension in Two Adult Horses. J Equine Vet Sci 2023;120:104193.

44. Mair TS, Pearson GR, Scase TJ. Multiple small intestinal pseudodiverticula associated with lymphoma in three horses. Equine Vet J 2011;39:128–32.

45. Acevedo HD, Hassebroek AM, Leventhal HR, et al. Colonic T-cell–rich, large B-cell lymphoma associated with equid herpesvirus 5 infection and secondary trans-colonic fistula in a horse. J Vet Diagn Invest 2023;3:272–7.

46. Cabral FC, Krajewski KM, Kim KW, et al. Peritoneal lymphomatosis: CT and PET/CT findings and how to differentiate between carcinomatosis and sarcomatosis. Cancer Imag 2013;2:162–70.

47. Roberts MC, Pinsent PJN. Malabsorption in the Horse associated with Alimentary Lymphosarcoma. Equine Vet J 1975l;3:166–72.

48. Zimmerman B, Jones S, Rotstein DS. Large granular lymphoma in a mule. Vet Rec 2004;15:462–3.

49. Platt H. Alimentary lymphoma in the horse. J Comp Pathol 1987;97(1):1–10.

50. Sharma D, Subbarao G, Saxena R. Hepatoblastoma. Semin Diagn Pathol 2017; 34:192–200.

51. Luethy D, Frimberger AE, Bedenice D, et al. Retrospective evaluation of clinical outcome after chemotherapy for lymphoma in 15 equids (1991-2017). J Vet Intern Med 2019;2:953–60.

52. Théon AP, Pusterla N, Magdesian KG, et al. Phase I Dose Escalation of Doxorubicin Chemotherapy in Tumor-Bearing Equidae. J Vet Intern Med 2013;5: 1209–17.

53. Théon AP, Pusterla N, Magdesian KG, et al. A Pilot Phase II Study of the Efficacy and Biosafety of Doxorubicin Chemotherapy in Tumor-Bearing Equidae. J Vet Intern Med 2013;6:1581–8.

54. Dabareiner RM, Goodrich LR, Sullins KE. Large colon resection for treatment of lymphosarcoma in two horses. J Am Vet Med Assoc 1996;6:895–7.

55. Fulton IC, Brown CM, Yamini B. Adenocarcinoma of intestinal origin in a horse: diagnosis by abdominocentesis and laparoscopy. Equine Vet J 1990;6:447–8.

56. Jann HW, Breshears MA, Allison RW, et al. Occult metastatic intestinal adenocarcinoma resulting in pathological fracture of the proximal humerus. Equine Vet J 2009;9:915–7.

57. Kirchhof N, Steinhauer D, Fey K. Equine adenocarcinomas of the large intestine with osseous metaplasia. J Comp Pathol 1996;4:451–6.

58. Roy MF, Parente EJ, Donaldson MT, et al. Successful treatment of a colonic adenocarcinoma in a horse. Equine Vet J 2010;1:102–4.

59. Wright JA, Edwards GB. Adenocarcinoma of the intestine in a horse: An unusual occurrence. Equine Vet J 1984;2:136–7.

60. Muñoz MJA, Lemberger K, Cadoré JL, et al. Small Intestine Adenocarcinoma in Conjunction with Multiple Adenomas Causing Acute Colic in a Horse. J Vet Diagn Invest 2008;1:121–4.
61. Livesey MA, Hulland TJ, Yovich JV. Colic in two horses associated with smooth muscle intestinal tumours. Equine Vet J 1986;4:334–7.
62. Mair TS, Taylor FGR, Brown PJ. Leiomyosarcoma of the Duodenum in two Horses. J Comp Pathol 1990;1:119–23.
63. Watt BC, Trostle SS, Cooley AJ. Intraluminal leiomyoma colon polyp in a mare. Equine Vet J 2001;3:326–8.
64. Oreff GL, Tatz AJ, Dahan R, et al. Successful removal of jejunal leiomyosarcoma in a Quarter Horse mare. Equine Vet Educ 2018;11:458–62.
65. Müller AC, Onkels AK, Köhler K, et al. Equine gastrointestinal stromal tumours (GISTs) of the small intestine as cause of acute colic: Pferdeheilkunde Equine. Med 2021;5:474–80.
66. Stephan S, Hug S, Hilbe M. Gastrointestinal Stromal Tumor in the Cecum of a Horse. Case Rep Vet Med 2012;1–5.
67. Hafner S, Harmon BG, King T. Gastrointestinal Stromal Tumors of the Equine Cecum. Vet Pathol 2001 Mar;2:242–6.
68. Kirchhof N, Scheidemann W, Baumgärtner W. Multiple Peripheral Nerve Sheath Tumors in the Small Intestine of a Horse. Vet Pathol 1996 Nov;6:727–30.
69. Southwood L. Disseminated Hemangiosarcoma in the Horse: 35 Cases. J Vet Intern Med 2000;14:105–9.
70. Allen D, Swayne D, Belknap JK. Ganglioneuroma as a cause of small intestinal obstruction in the horse: A case report. Cornell Vet 1989;2:133–41.
71. MacGillivray KC, Sweeney RW, Piero FD. Metastatic Melanoma in Horses. J Vet Intern Med 2002;4:452–6.
72. Linnenkohl W, Mair T, Fews D. Case report of atypical infiltrative lipomatosis of the equine mesojejunum: Lipomatosis of the equine mesojejunum. Equine Vet Educ 2013;5:237–40.
73. Henry GA, Yamini B. Equine Colonic Lipomatosis. J Vet Diagn Invest 1995;4: 578–80.
74. Lesca H, Fairburn A, Fitzharris LE, et al. Ultrasonographic identification of mesenteric lipomatosis in a Shetland mare with recurrent colic episodes. Equine Vet Educ 2023;3:186–92.
75. Riley E, Martindale A, Maran B, et al. Small colon lipomatosis resulting in refractory small colon impaction in a Tennessee Walking Horse. Equine Vet Educ 2007; 9:484–7.
76. De Bont MP, Malbon AJ, Sardon D, et al. Caecal lipomatosis as a cause of colic in a 9-year-old gelding: Caecal lipomatosis as a cause of colic. Equine Vet Educ 2013;5:241–4.
77. Head KW, Else RW, Dubielzig RR. Tumors of the alimentary tract. Tumors Domest Anim 2002;4:477–8.
78. Dobromylskyj MJ, Copas V, Durham A, et al. Disseminated lipid-rich peritoneal mesothelioma in a horse. J Vet Diagn Invest 2011;3:615–8.
79. Passantino G, Sassi E, Filippi I, et al. Thoracic and Abdominal Mesothelioma in an Older Horse in Lazio Region. Animals 2022;19:1–10.
80. Stoica G, Cohen N, Mendes O, et al. Use of Immunohistochemical Marker Calretinin in the Diagnosis of a Diffuse Malignant Metastatic Mesothelioma in an Equine. J Vet Diagn Invest 2004;3:240–3.
81. Ricketts SW, Peace CK. A Case of Peritoneal Mesothelioma in a Thoroughbred Mare. Equine Vet J 1976;2:78–80.

82. Rendle DI, Hewetson M, Barron R, et al. Tachypnoea and pleural effusion in a mare with metastatic pancreatic adenocarcinoma. Vet Rec 2006;11:356–8.
83. Ruby RE. Malignant glucagonoma associated with hyperglycaemia, hypertriglyceridaemia, Candidiasis and bacterial pneumonia in a 12-year-old Arabian gelding. Equine Vet Educ 2020;11:309–12.
84. Beeler-Marfisi J, Arroyo L, Caswell JL, et al. Equine Primary Liver Tumors: A Case Series and Review of the Literature. J Vet Diagn Invest 2010;2:174–83.
85. Cantile C, Arispici M, Abramo F, et al. Hepatoblastoma in a foal. Equine Vet J 2001;2:214–6.
86. Neu SM. Hepatoblastoma in an Equine Fetus. J Vet Diagn Invest 1993;4:634–7.
87. Jeffcott LB. Primary liver-cell carcinoma in a young thoroughbred horse. J Pathol 1969;2:394–7.
88. Lopez B. and Epstein K., Cholangiocarcinoma Comparative Veterinary Anatomy: A Clinical Approach, First Edition, Academic Press; London, England, 763–770.
89. Conti MB. Clinical findings and diagnosis in a case of cholangiocellular carcinoma in a horse. Vet Res Commun 2008;1:271–3.
90. Axon J, Russell C, Begg A, et al. Erythrocytosis and pleural effusion associated with a hepatoblastoma in a Thoroughbred yearling. Aust Vet J 2008;8:329–33.
91. Tirosh-Levy S, Perl S, Valentine BA, et al. Erythrocytosis and fatigue fractures associated with hepatoblastoma in a 3-year-old gelding. J S Afr Vet Assoc 2019;0:1–5.
92. De Vries C, Vanhaesebrouck E, Govaere, et al. Congenital Ascites due to Hepatoblastoma with Extensive Peritoneal Implantation Metastases in a Premature Equine Fetus. J Comp Pathol 2013;2–3:214–9.
93. Kato M. Combined hepatocellular carcinoma and cholangiocarcinoma in a mare. J Comp Pathol 1997;4:409–13.
94. Salvaggio A. Hepatic Biliary Adenofibroma: A Hitherto Unrecognized Tumor in Equines. Report of a Case 2003;1:114–6.
95. Brown DL. Mesenchymal Hamartoma of the Liver in a Late-Term Equine Fetus. Veterinary Pathology 2007;1:100–2.
96. Roperto F. Mixed hamartoma of the liver in an equine foetus. Equine Vet J 1984;1: 218–20.

Tumors of the Urogenital Tract

Jamie Prutton, BSc (Hons), BVSc, MBA, CMgr, MCMI, MRCVS[a],[*],
Rachel Tucker, BSc, BVetMed, MVetMed, CertAVP(ESO), MRCVS[b]

KEYWORDS

• Equine • Urogenital • Oncology • Tumor • Neoplasia • Penis • Prepuce

KEY POINTS

- Neoplasia of the urogenital tract is relatively uncommon; squamous cell carcinoma of the external genitalia is the most frequently seen.
- There is no current evidence for systemic chemotherapeutics in urogenital neoplasia but topical chemotherapeutics have been reported for some cases.
- Surgical procedures can be curative although the location of the tumor can make treatment impossible.
- Prognosis is often hard to give due to the paucity of reports.

INTRODUCTION

Neoplasia has been reported to involve the majority of the urinary system of the horse, with tumors affecting the kidneys and bladder most comprehensively described. Primary tumors of the external genitalia are relatively common in the horse and are easily identified on clinical examination, whilst primary tumors of the upper urogenital tract are uncommon. This article will highlight the common tumors, their clinical presentations, and discuss potential medical and surgical treatment options available. The less common neoplasms will be mentioned but not discussed in depth.

DISCUSSION
Renal Neoplasia

Renal neoplasms have historically been considered to be metastases; however, a more recent retrospective study found primary disease to be the cause of renal neoplasia in 15 out of 20 cases.[1] Renal neoplasia is most likely to be unilateral but in rare instances, can be bilateral.

[a] Equine Internal Medicine, Liphook Equine Hospital, Forest Mere, Liphook, Hampshire GU30 7JG, UK; [b] Equine Surgery, Liphook Equine Hospital, Forest Mere, Liphook, Hampshire GU30 7JG, UK
[*] Corresponding author.
E-mail address: Jamie.Prutton@theleh.co.uk

Vet Clin Equine 40 (2024) 487–499
https://doi.org/10.1016/j.cveq.2024.07.012
0749-0739/24/© 2024 Elsevier Inc. All rights reserved, including those for text and data mining, AI training, and similar technologies.
vetequine.theclinics.com

Clinical symptoms of renal neoplasia are often nonspecific, with horses presenting for poor performance, lethargy, acute or chronic weight loss, fever, and recurrent colic. More specific signs can include hematuria, ascites, stranguria (if there is discomfort associated with urination), or in some cases polyuria and polydipsia.[2]

When renal neoplasia is considered a differential diagnosis, diagnostic investigation should commence with rectal palpation of relevant accessible structures, trans-abdominal (**Fig. 1**) and rectal ultrasound, urinalysis, hematology, and biochemistry. Blood sampling may reveal biochemical changes associated with renal dysfunction; elevated creatinine, elevated urea, anemia, elevated symmetric dimethylarginine (SDMA), hypoalbuminaemia, and electrolyte abnormalities.[3] It is important to note that serum creatinine often remains within reference range if neoplasia is only affecting 1 kidney due to the ability of the normal kidney to compensate and excrete creatinine.

Cystoscopy allows for visual assessment of the urethra, bladder, and ureteral openings for tumors that are present within the mucosa or protruding into the bladder. It also enables sterile urine collection from the bladder and from the ureters if a secondary infection is considered a concern. Sampling from the ureters must be performed with care to avoid iatrogenic trauma and consequent blood contamination of the urine sample which could confuse their interpretation if attempting to work out which kidney is affected. Air used to inflate the bladder should be removed after the procedure due to a report of fatal air embolism occurring during a cystoscopy[4] although the risk is very small. Trans-endoscopic pinch biopsies can be taken of the bladder mucosa although neoplasia may erroneously be diagnosed in inflammatory disease states due to dysplastic cells[5] (**Fig. 2**). Therefore, care should be taken when interpreting these results although many samples in the study (7/8) were definitively neoplastic and therefore the technique has a place in diagnostics.

Renal biopsy can be performed percutaneously under ultrasound guidance using a Trucut needle or automated biopsy instrument. The procedure is associated with a risk of morbidity and mortality, primarily that of hemorrhage, and it is therefore prudent to assess hematology and clotting times prior to biopsy. Renal biopsies in 151 horses were reported, 94% of the samples were suitable for diagnostic analysis and 20/28 (71%) of biopsy findings correlated with a postmortem diagnosis.[6] There were only 4 diagnoses of neoplasia in the cohort. The complication rate was 11.3%, due to hemorrhage, colic, or pyrexia. One fatality was recorded due to exsanguination into the

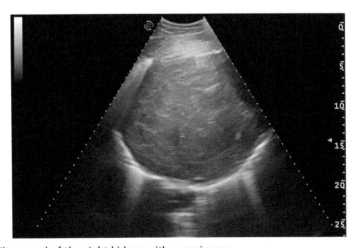

Fig. 1. Ultrasound of the right kidney with a carcinoma.

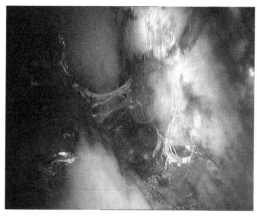

Fig. 2. Cystoscopy showing ulcerative cystitis that, on biopsy, showed evidence of dysplastic cells.

abdominal cavity post biopsy. Therefore, clients should be advised of the risks before the procedure is performed.

Multiple single case studies exist for renal and bladder tumors but there are few retrospective studies. A review of 1069 postmortem examinations identified 20 cases of renal neoplasia, giving a prevalence of 1.87% in a mixed population of horses/ponies.[1] Primary neoplasia comprised carcinoma (9/15), adenoma (4/15), renal neuroendocrine (1/15), and nephroblastoma (1/15). Secondary renal neoplasia was identified with lymphosarcoma (3/5) being predominant, a melanoma, and a hemangiosarcoma. A range of breeds of horse and pony were represented and all were over 10 yrs old. There were no consistent presenting clinical signs to indicate renal neoplasia although 2 carcinomas presented with severe hemoabdomen due to rupture of the renal capsule.

Twenty seven cases of renal carcinoma were presented, with Thoroughbreds and geldings being over represented, although there was no age effect.[7] Routine laboratory analyses were unremarkable with no evidence of renal dysfunction. Urinalysis and peritoneal fluid were abnormal but the changes were nonspecific. Ultrasound was found to be the most useful technique in identifying and characterizing abnormal renal tissue. Definitive pre-mortem diagnosis was made on biopsy in 7 cases. Distant metastases were identified in 19/27 cases, highlighting the importance of tumor staging. Twenty five of 27 cases were not discharged following presentation and only 1 horse survived to 1 year following diagnosis.

Three cases of primary renal hemangiosarcoma all of which presented with insidious weight loss and one presented with terminal epistaxis and abdominal pain have been described.[8] All 3 cases were euthanised. Thirty-five cases of hemangiosarcoma were reported in the horse where there was only 1 primary renal hemangiosarcoma but 9 cases with metatstatic hemangiosarcoma within the kidney.[9]

Prognosis and treatment

In cases of renal neoplasia, the prognosis is grave with most cases euthanased due to severity of signs at presentation and lack of treatment options. Chemotherapy has not been described.

Nephrectomy is occasionally indicated for treatment of unilateral renal neoplasia when there is no evidence of metastatic spread and when sufficient contralateral renal function has been established. The kidneys sit dorsally in the retroperitoneal space making nephrectomy technically challenging due to the limited surgical exposure achievable. A neoplastic kidney may be much enlarged, and local invasion of surrounding structures such as the caudal vena cava is possible. Not all cases are operable.[7] In the anesthetized horse, the kidney is exposed via a transcostal approach, or via ventral midline incision in smaller animals. There is a trend toward standing laparoscopic nephrectomy, avoiding the need for general anesthesia and rib resection, providing superior visual control of ligation and transection, and a shorter recovery.[10] Laparoscopic surgery with mini laparotomy or hand-assisted laparoscopy is described.[11,12]

Bladder Neoplasia

Neoplasms of the bladder are very rare in the equine patient. They may be highly malignant, although slow growing, with metastases likely occurring most commonly in the peritoneum, liver, and lungs.[13] Neoplasms seen in the bladder include squamous cell carcinoma, transitional cell carcinoma, and botryoid rhabdomyosarcoma.[5,14,15] Benign tumors can occur and include papilloma, adenoma, fibroma, leiomyoma, angioma, and polyps.[16,17]

Hematuria is the most common clinical finding in these cases and ultrasound and cystoscopy are considered the main diagnostic modalities. Common differential diagnoses include urolithiasis and cystitis. It is important to note that idiopathic hemorrhagic cystitis can appear grossly and histopathologically as neoplasia but responds well to medical management.[5]

Clinical signs tend to occur late in the course of disease, limiting treatment options due to the advanced state (size/infiltration) of the primary tumor and the presence of metastasis. Additionally, these tumors do not respond well to cytotoxic agents and surgical access is limited. Chemotherapy alone has been attempted unsuccessfully[16,18] and tried with limited success alongside mass resection or debulking surgery. Treatment with cyclooxygenase 2 (COX-2), selective nonsteroidal anti-inflammatory medication, has been tried, with euthanasia required after 1 month of treatment in a single case of transitional cell carcinoma.[19] Successful treatment was reported following surgical debulking and piroxicam therapy in a case of transitional cell carcinoma.[14]

Open surgical access to the bladder is challenging, due to its anatomic location within the pelvic cavity. Even if accessible, complete mass resection may be impossible due to the lesion size and depth of penetration into the bladder wall. The bladder is accessible laparoscopically; however, laparoscopic treatment of bladder neoplasia has not yet been established. Partial cystoplasty has been reported via an open abdominal approach for successful removal of a mass from the dorso-cranial portion of the bladder which was confirmed as squamous cell carcinoma.[20] It might be possible to remove mucosal tumors utilizing endoscopic laser, but this has not been reported.

Other neoplasia

No tumors of the urethra have been reported whilst a single case of ureteral transitional cell carcinoma is described.[21]

MALE REPRODUCTIVE SYSTEM
Penis and Prepuce

Penial and preputial neoplasms are relatively common and are the most frequently reported neoplasia of the male reproductive tract.[22] Accessory sex gland neoplasia is very uncommon with 1 reported case series (n = 2) of adenocarcinoma diagnosed on postmortem.[23] Finally, the scrotum is subject to all the neoplasms of the epidermis and therefore will not be discussed.

Clinical signs associated with neoplasms of the penis and prepuce are primarily noted due to visually abnormal tissue. Visual inspection of tumors on the external genitalia can generally guide the clinician toward the likely cause although histopathology should always be undertaken to confirm the diagnosis and the extent of local infiltration of tissues. For example, squamous cell carcinoma (SCC) precancerous (solar elastosis) lesions will appear as areas of depigmentation, although carcinoma in situ and papilloma can appear similarly. Early lesions appear as small, slightly raised, reddened plaques and may be single or multiple. Advanced lesions appear as florid, cauliflower-like masses with areas of necrosis and hemorrhage. Alongside a mass or visible lesion, in SCC cases, purulent or sanguinous discharge may be noted (42%) with impaired micturition sometimes occurring (22%).[24] Occasionally, there may be pruritis, wide base stance, or altered hindlimb gait. Masses may be missed until these secondary events occur as the lesion itself is not always externally visible.

Diagnostic evaluation must involve inspection of the entire penis/prepuce which routinely requires the administration of acepromazine and sedation to facilitate the penis dropping and subsequent cleaning. Appropriate preparation for visual inspection allows the size, location, number, and potentially degree of infiltration of the neoplasms to be noted.

Assessment of the local lymph nodes should be undertaken as metastases do occur. The superficial inguinal lymph nodes lie dorsolateral to the penis or mammary glands and the deep inguinal lymph nodes are located just outside the pelvis adjacent to the internal inguinal ring. The medial iliac lymph nodes (adjacent to the external iliac arteries) can be evaluated per rectum. If lymph node palpation is abnormal, biopsy should be considered where lymph nodes are safely accessible, using a Trucut needle as fine needle aspirates can result in both false-positive and false-negative results making interpretation very difficult.[25] It should be considered that although regional lymphadenopathy may be an indicator of metastases, enlargement can also be due to "eactive" lymph nodes, secondary to concomitant inflammation or infection. When assessing lymph nodes, 34% (28/82) of the penile SCC had inguinal lymph node enlargement but only 9/28 of those horses had neoplasia confirmed by histopathology, but 9% of normal lymph nodes were also found to contain neoplastic cells.[24]

Thoracic radiography and abdominal ultrasound should be considered part of the diagnostic evaluation of cases although frequently it does not confirm any abnormalities. Nodular masses were reported within the thorax in 1 of 27 horses with penile squamous cell carcinoma and this horse was alive after 4 years following resection of the primary tumor bringing into question the relevance of the findings.[24]

Biopsy and histopathology are useful to guide the treatment plan. Histopathology can guide prognosis as poorly differentiated neoplasms are more likely to metastasize, warranting more radical resection.[26] It should be noted that inflammatory conditions of the penis are relatively common and therefore biopsy can highlight differentials such as granulomatous lesions, infection, or Habronema.

Any tumors of epithelial or mesenchymal origin can affect the male external genitalia. The most commonly described tumor is squamous cell carcinoma,[22,27,28] followed by papilloma, melanoma, and sarcoid. Rarely reported diagnoses include hemangioma, basal cell carcinoma, neurofibrosarcoma, adenocarcinoma, and fibrosarcoma. External genitalia neoplasms are 12.1 times (95% CI, 9.8–15.0) as likely to be SCC, compared with any other tumor (excluding papillomas).[28]

Neoplasia of the penis and prepuce most commonly affects older horses, with a reported mean age of 19.5 years (8–33 years), with no SCC case in horses under 13 years.[24] More specifically, the mean age of horses with SCC to be 16.4 years.[28] There is no specific breed predilection although ponies and cobs are overrepresented and thoroughbreds underrepresented. Breeds with decreased skin and hair pigmentation are thought to be predisposed for the development of SCC[29,30] although it is not clear if this is relevant to the penis where ultraviolet exposure is low. Most literature pertains to the relative increase in SCC seen in geldings versus stallions but the biased population of equids may affect these results.

Multiple potential etiologies for SCC have been discussed in the literature. Smegma may help propagate the disease, act as a nidus for infection, and may be pro-inflammatory but has not been shown to be carcinogenic. In humans, SCC of the cervix is nearly always associated with human papilloma virus, and in equids Equus, caballus papilloma virus 2 (EcPV-2) and subsequent transformation of papilloma to SCC might be implicated. EcPV-2 has been identified in SCC with a frequency ranging from 43% to 90% of genital SCC although penile tissues of horses without SCC were also positive for EcPV-2 (5%–10%).[31–35] Therefore, it seems likely that EcPV-2 plays a role in the pathology of SCC.

Primary treatment for penial or preputial SCC is surgical resection although early, precancerous, or solar elastosis lesions may be amenable to topical chemotherapy. Medical therapy can be utilized for superficial SCC. 5-Fluoruracil (5-FU) topically had a success rate of 10/11 cases with the product being applied to mares daily for 2 weeks then every 2 weeks thereafter and for males applied every 14 days. The remission was 7 months to 52 months depending on the follow-up period.[36] Intralesional 5-FU was only successful at reducing tumor size in 5 cases rather than inducing remission and therefore is not advised.[37]

Various other medical therapies have been reported for SCC in other anatomic locations but not within the urogenital tract and include photodynamic therapy with verteporfin following excision of the mass[38]; metronomic therapy with meloxicam and cyclophosphamide; and immunotherapy and adjunctive intralesional chemotherapy with cisplatin, bleomycin, 5-FU, and mitomycin C.

The goal of surgery is to remove the tumor with sufficient margins to prevent recurrence and is performed in most cases in the anesthetized horse. A range of surgical methods are described, and the choice of procedure depends on location and local extent of neoplasia and amount of surgical margin desired. Surgical options include local mass excision, segmental posthetomy (reefing), distal phallectomy, and en-bloc resection of the penis and prepuce.

Segmental posthetomy removes a circumferential cuff of the preputial lamina. It is most applicable when the lesion(s) is thought to not involve the tunica albuginea. Distal phallectomy is applicable when only the distal penis is affected. It can be performed in combination with segmental posthetomy if required. Various techniques of phallectomy have been described. Creation of a triangular urethrostomy with the base of the triangle positioned distally reduces the risk of urethral stricture.[30,39] Standing distal phallectomy has been described whereby the distal penis was sharply transected distal to a purpose made tourniquet with no additional surgical closure. The tourniquet was left in situ to slough with the distal tissue. All 11 horses were reported to appear comfortable following surgery. En bloc resection allows removal of the entire free portion of the penis, the internal and external lamina of the prepuce, and potentially the regional lymph nodes. The new urethral opening may be created at the level of amputation in the caudal ventral abdomen[40] or with retroversion of the remaining distal penis to a vertical subischial location[41] or without retroversion to leave a redundant section of distal penis in situ.[42] An optimum method is not known; however, a subishial vertical urethrostomy enables greater margins to be achieved. Histopathology of resected tissue is strongly advised to establish whether clear margins have been obtained.

Postoperative complications are more frequently encountered with radical resection techniques, including hematuria, wound healing complications, postoperative pain, and laminitis.[42,43] Accurate surgery, diligent postoperative monitoring, and proactive multimodal analgesia is advised to minimize these occurrences.

Survival rates are difficult to compare due to differences in reporting techniques. SCC survival rates vary and have been reported as: 64.5% survival without recurrence for up to at 18+ months[44]; 81% survival without recurrence at 12+ months[45]; 70.5% non-recurrence at 18 months; a 74.4% non-recurrence following partial phallectomy; and an 87.5% non-recurrence following en-bloc resection.[24] Therefore, it appears that more radical resection techniques are associated with a lower recurrence rate but a higher short-term post operative morbidity rate.

Testicles

Reports of testicular neoplasia are rare and are most often individual case reports. Tumors can be separated into 3 groups: germinal tumors (seminoma, teratoma, carcinoma, and embryonic carcinoma); non-germinal tumors (Leydig [interstitial] cell, Sertoli [sustentacular] cell, mast cell and lipoma), and other cell origin tumors (leiomyoma, mast cell tumor). Published reports confirm tumors are seen in both descended and cryptochid testicles[46] although there is an increased frequency of cryptorchidism and testicular tumors, particularly teratoma. Therefore, appropriate surgical removal of retained testicular tissue should be undertaken when a cryptorchidism is suspected.

Clinically, horses will present with enlargement of a testicle and treatment relies on orchidectomy of the affected testicle. This is frequently curative and cases of primary testicular neoplasia with secondary metastases have not been reported. Ultrasound with biopsy will be diagnostic and ensure that the enlargement is neoplastic rather than inflammatory. There are no reports of chemotherapy being used in testicular neoplasia.

NEOPLASIA OF THE FEMALE REPRODUCTIVE TRACT
Vulva and Vagina

Much like the male reproductive tract, the external genitalia of females are most frequently affected but neoplasms of the uterus and ovaries are also reported.[47]

There are several single or small case reports of squamous cell carcinoma affecting the vulva and vagina but no larger scale studies[48] (**Fig. 3**). Other tumors reported to affect the external genitalia include hemangiosarcoma and solar elastoses,[49] leiomyosarcoma,[50] melanoma,[51] and apocrine carcinoma.[52] Vulva papillomatosis and carcinoma in situ was described in a 25-year-old mare affecting the commissures of vulva and vestibule walls which was treated by surgical debulking with a diode laser and 3 treatments with 5-FU, followed by further laser resection 5 months later.[53] There was no recurrence after a further 4 months. Two additional cases of squamous cell carcinoma of the labia, vulva, and vestibule are reported and were treated by surgical excision without recurrence at 1 year.[48,54]

Diagnosis and medical management of SCC of the vulva is most likely the same as for penile and preputial SCC, given the paucity of published information.

Uterus

Uterine tumors are rare in horses with sparse individual case reports. Uterine neoplasia may be associated with infertility, abdominal pain, bloody vulvar discharge[55] or may be an incidental finding. Leiomyoma, a benign neoplasia of the smooth muscle, is the most commonly reported uterine tumor in 10% to 50% of uterine tumors.[47] Leiomyosarcoma,

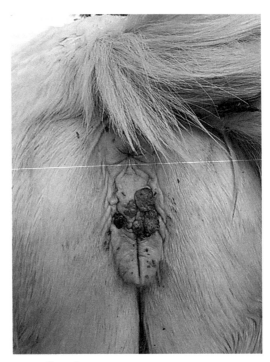

Fig. 3. Vulval squamous cell carcinoma.

adenocarcinoma, and fibroma are also reported.[16,56,57] A familial pattern for both uterine leiomyomas and fibromas has been suggested.[58] Non-neoplastic causes of these presenting signs should also be considered.

Diagnosis of uterine tumors can be performed via rectal ultrasound and hysteroscopy. Subsequently endometrial biopsy may aid in assessment of uterine health but is unlikely to be valuable for tumor diagnosis due to the relatively superficial nature of the technique.

Surgery has been reported for leiomyoma where it is typically a solitary well circumscribed mass, involving the myometrium. Hysterotomy and mass removal or partial hysterectomy may be performed and can preserve fertility. The surgical approach will depend on the location of the mass, with paramedian approach under general anesthesia (GA) and standing hand-assisted laparoscopic surgery described.[59–61] The maximum amount of a uterine horn that can be removed and still result in pregnancy is unknown, but 1 successful pregnancy with full-term gestation was achieved after 50% of 1 horn had been removed.[61] Alternatively, ovariohysterectomy may be indicated which can be performed in its entirety under GA via a caudal ventral midline incision.[62,63] Significant postop morbidity resulted in euthanasia in one mare was euthanised secondary to postoperative peritonitis. Ovariohysterectomy can also be performed in a 2-step procedure whereby the mesovarium and mesometrium are transected via a laparoscopic procedure in the standing horse[64] or in the anesthetized horse followed by a caudal ventral midline incision under GA to allow transection of the uterine body and removal from the abdomen.[65] The challenge for complete ovariohysterectomy is to remove as much uterus as possible while minimizing abdominal contamination at surgery.

No medical managemental techniques are reported for uterine tumors.

Ovaries

Granulosa cell tumors (GCT) are the most common tumor of the equine ovary[66,67] and arise from the granulosa-theca cells. The mean age of mares with a GCT was 11 ±5 years[67] although reports exist in foals.[68] There is no breed predilection. Although frequently unilateral, the tumor can be bilateral. The tumor completely obliterates the affected ovary giving a typical diagnostic image on ultrasound and hormone profile. The hormone profile includes increases in testosterone and inhibin which will lead to the clinical behavioral changes. Other ovarian tumors that have been reported as single case reports include cystadenoma, cystadenocarcinoma, teratoma, teratocarcinoma, dysgerminoma, and lymphoma.

Mares with GCTs will often present with abnormal behavior such as stallion-like behavior (54%), aggression (31%), prolonged oestrus/nymphomania (19%), and anoestrus (8%).[67] Diagnostic confirmation of a GCT is via both ultrasound, which shows a multicystic or "honeycomb" appearance of the ovary, and serum anti-Mullerian hormone.[69] Historically, variations in testosterone, inhibin, and progesterone were used but these have become obsolete. Most cases are unilateral with only 27% (14/52) patients having bilateral GCTs.[67]

Surgery is the treatment of choice for GCTs and is curative. Surgery can be performed by colpotomy,[70] flank, paramedian, or a ventral midline celiotomy,[71,72] or more recently via flank laparoscopy.[73] In the most recent study of 52 cases, 73% underwent standing laparoscopic procedure with the remaining being performed under GA. When surgery is performed, 94% of the cases discharged with laparoscopic ovariectomies had a complication rate of 34% but this was lower than other techniques performed under general anesthesia (40%–63%).[67] Long-term complications were uncommon (11%). More recently, severe hemoperitoneum has been reported during the surgical procedure.[74]

No medical management exists for GCTs in the mare.

SUMMARY

Medical management of neoplasms in equids is poorly reported and this is especially true for those of the urogenital tract. Topical treatments should be considered in cases of small, early squamous cell carcinoma or the external genitalia otherwise surgery will often be the primary treatment modality.

Diagnosis and confirmation of the neoplasia warrants a thorough evaluation including ultrasound, endoscopy, hematological analysis, and biopsy. With this complete picture, advise can be given for the prognosis although exact numbers for most neoplasms are unknown.

Given the rarity of these neoplasms, it seems unlikely that large number case series will be created to further guide treatment and prognosis.

CLINICS CARE POINTS

- Prompt evaluation and treatment of suspected neoplasia is required to optimise clinical outcome.
- Discuss cases early with surgeons to decide if surgical intervention is appropriate.

DISCLOSURE

The authors have nothing to disclose.

REFERENCES

1. Vienenkötter J, Siudak K, Stallenberger L, et al. Renal neoplasia in horses – a retrospective study. Tierarztl Prax Ausg G 2017;45(05):290–5.
2. Birkmann K, Trump M, Dettwiler M, et al. Severe polyuria and polydipsia as major clinical signs in a horse with unilateral renal adenocarcinoma. Equine Vet Educ 2016;28(12):675–80.
3. Gratwick Z. An updated review: Laboratory investigation of equine renal disease. Equine Vet Educ 2021;33(10):546–55.
4. Gordon E, Schlipf JW, Husby KA, et al. Two occurrences of presumptive venous air embolism in a gelding during cystoscopy and perineal urethrotomy. Equine Vet Educ 2017;29(5):236–41.
5. Smith FL, Magdesian KG, Michel AO, et al. Equine idiopathic hemorrhagic cystitis: Clinical features and comparison with bladder neoplasia. Veterinary Internal Medicine 2018;32(3):1202–9.
6. Tyner GA, Nolen-Walston RD, Hall T, et al. A Multicenter Retrospective Study of 151 Renal Biopsies in Horses. Veterinary Internal Medicne 2011;25(3):532–9.
7. Wise LN, Bryan JN, Sellon DC, et al. A Retrospective Analysis of Renal Carcinoma in the Horse. Veterinary Internal Medicne 2009;23(4):913–8.
8. Hughes K, Scott VHL, Blanck M, et al. Equine renal hemangiosarcoma: clinical presentation, pathologic features, and pSTAT3 expression. J Vet Diagn Invest 2018; 30(2):268–74.
9. Southwood LL, Schott HC, Henry CJ, et al. Disseminated Hemangiosarcoma in the Horse: 35 Cases. Veterinary Internal Medicne 2000;14(1):105–9.
10. Mariën T. Laparoscopic nephrectomy in the standing horse. In: Fischer AT, editor. Equine diagnostic surgical laparoscopy. Philadelphia: Saunders; 2002. p. 273–81.
11. Röcken M, Mosel G, Stehle C, et al. Left- and Right-Sided Laparoscopic-Assisted Nephrectomy in Standing Horses with Unilateral Renal Disease. Vet Surg 2007; 36(6):568–72.
12. Ragle CA. In: Advances in equine laparoscopy. John Wiley & Sons; 2012. Available at: https://books.google.com/books?hl=en&lr=&id=flwqtBSnKUgC&oi=fnd& pg=PR9&dq=Nephrectomy+In:+Advances+in+Equine+Laparoscopy+&ots=VL w5jbqqFJ&sig=pc3oONMb4S15ePfbYpeFzqFMD4Y. [Accessed 26 February 2024].
13. Patterson-Kane JC, Tramontin RR, Giles RC, et al. Transitional Cell Carcinoma of the Urinary Bladder in a Thoroughbred, with Intra-abdominal Dissemination. Vet Pathol 2000;37(6):692–5.
14. Lisowski ZM, Mair TS, Fews D. Transitional cell carcinoma of the urinary bladder in a 12-year-old Belgian Warmblood gelding. Equine Vet Educ 2015;27(7). https:// doi.org/10.1111/eve.12021.
15. Turnquist SE, Pace LW, Keegan K, et al. Botryoid Rhabdomyosarcoma of the Urinary Bladder in a Filly. J Vet Diagn Invest 1993;5(3):451–3.
16. Hurcombe SD, Slovis NM, Kohn CW, et al. Poorly differentiated leiomyosarcoma of the urogenital tract in a horse. J Am Vet Med Assoc 2008;233(12):1908–12.
17. Ricketts SW, Frauenfelder H, Button CJ, et al. Urinary retention in a pony gelding associated with a fibroepithelial polyp in the bladder. Equine Vet J 1983;15(2): 170–2.
18. Fischer AT, Spier S, Carlson GP, et al. Neoplasia of the equine urinary bladder as a cause of hematuria. J Am Vet Med Assoc 1985;186(12):1294–6.
19. Busechian S, Gialletti R, Brachelente C, et al. Transitional cell carcinoma of the bladder in a 12-year-old gelding. J Equine Vet Sci 2016;40:80–3.

20. Serena A, Naranjo C, Koch C, et al. Resection cystoplasty of a squamous cell carcinoma in a mare. Equine Vet Educ 2009;21(5):263–6.
21. Vercauteren G, Maes S, De Clercq D, et al. Ureteral Transitional Cell Carcinoma with Intra-abdominal and Distant Metastases in Two Horses. J Comp Pathol 2010; 143(4):340.
22. Brinsko SP. Neoplasia of the male reproductive tract. Vet Clin N Am Equine Pract 1998;14(3):517–33.
23. Knobbe M, Levine D, Habecker P, et al. Prostatic masses in geldings: two cases. J Equine Vet Sci 2012;32(10):628–33.
24. Van Den Top JGB, De Heer N, Klein WR, et al. Penile and preputial tumours in the horse: A retrospective study of 114 affected horses. Equine Vet J 2008;40(6): 528–32.
25. Van Den TOP JGB, Ensink JM, Gröne A, et al. Penile and preputial tumours in the horse: Literature review and proposal of a standardised approach. Equine Vet J 2010;42(8):746–57.
26. Van Den Top JGB, Harkema L, Lange C, et al. Expression of p53, Ki67, EcPV2- and EcPV3 DNA, and viral genes in relation to metastasis and outcome in equine penile and preputial squamous cell carcinoma. Equine Vet J 2015;47(2):188–95.
27. Van Den Top JGB, De Heer N, Klein WR, et al. Penile and preputial squamous cell carcinoma in the horse: A retrospective study of treatment of 77 affected horses. Equine Vet J 2008;40(6):533–7.
28. Schaffer PA, Wobeser B, Martin LER, et al. Cutaneous neoplastic lesions of equids in the central United States and Canada: 3,351 biopsy specimens from 3,272 equids (2000–2010). J Am Vet Med Assoc 2013;242(1):99–104.
29. Scott DW, Miller Jr WH. Squamous cell carcinoma. Equine Dermatology 2003;1: 707–12.
30. Schumacher J. Penis and prepuce. In: Auer JA, Stick JA, editors. Equine surgery. St Louis (MO): Elsevier; 2019. p. 1034–64.
31. Bogaert L, Willemsen A, Vanderstraeten E, et al. EcPV2 DNA in equine genital squamous cell carcinomas and normal genital mucosa. Vet Microbiol 2012; 158(1–2):33–41.
32. Knight CG, Munday JS, Peters J, et al. Equine Penile Squamous Cell Carcinomas Are Associated With the Presence of Equine Papillomavirus Type 2 DNA Sequences. Vet Pathol 2011;48(6):1190–4.
33. Newkirk KM, Hendrix DVH, Anis EA, et al. Detection of papillomavirus in equine periocular and penile squamous cell carcinoma. J Vet Diagn Invest 2014;26(1): 131–5.
34. Porcellato I, Mecocci S, Mechelli L, et al. Equine Penile Squamous Cell Carcinomas as a Model for Human Disease: A Preliminary Investigation on Tumor Immune Microenvironment. Cells 2020;9(11):2364.
35. Tuomisto L, Virtanen J, Kegler K, et al. Equus caballus papillomavirus type 2 (EcPV2)-associated benign penile lesions and squamous cell carcinomas. Veterinary Medicine Science 2024;10(1):e1342.
36. Fortier LA, MacHarg MA. Topical use of 5-fluorouracil for treatment of squamous cell carcinoma of the external genitalia of horses: 11 cases (1988-1992). J Am Vet Med Assoc 1994;205:1183.
37. Pucket JD, Gilmour MA. Intralesional 5-fluorouracil (5-FU) for the treatment of eyelid squamous cell carcinoma in 5 horses. Equine Vet Educ 2014;26(6):331–5.
38. Giuliano EA, Johnson PJ, Delgado C, et al. Local photodynamic therapy delays recurrence of equine periocular squamous cell carcinoma compared to cryotherapy. Vet Ophthalmol 2014;17(s1):37–45.

39. Williams ZJ, French S, Hollinger C, et al. Antemortem diagnosis of renal haemangiosarcoma in a Hanoverian gelding. Equine Vet Educ 2024;36(3). https://doi.org/10.1111/eve.13895.
40. Doles J, Williams JW, Yarbrough TB. Penile Amputation and Sheath Ablation in the Horse. Vet Surg 2001;30(4):327–31.
41. Archer DC, Edwards GB. En bloc resection of the penis in five geldings. Equine Vet Educ 2010;16(1):12–9.
42. Wylie CE, Payne RJ. A modified surgical technique for penile amputation and preputial ablation in the horse. Equine Vet Educ 2016;28(5):269–75.
43. Tucker R, South V, Robinson N, et al. Increased risk of fatal laminitis during hospitalisation amongst phallectomy patients compared to laparotomy patients in a UK equine hospital over 10 years. Equine Vet J 2023;55(S58):22–3.
44. Howarth S, Lucke VM, Pearson H. Squamous cell carcinoma of the equine external genitalia: a review and assessment of penile amputation and urethrostomy as a surgical treatment. Equine Vet J 1991;23(1):53–8.
45. Mair TS, Walmsley JP, Phillips TJ. Surgical treatment of 45 horses affected by squamous cell carcinoma of the penis and prepuce. Equine Vet J 2000;32(5):406–10.
46. Valentine BA. Equine testicular tumours. Equine Vet Educ 2009;21(4):177–8.
47. McCue PM. Neoplasia of the female reproductive tract. Vet Clin N Am Equine Pract 1998;14(3):505–15.
48. Raś A, Otrocka-Domagała I, Raś-Noryńska M. Two different clinical forms of squamous cell carcinoma (SCC) in the perineum and vulva of two mares. BMC Vet Res 2020;16(1):464.
49. Gumber S, Baia P, Wakamatsu N. Vulvar epithelioid hemangiosarcoma with solar elastosis in a mare. J Vet Diagn Invest 2011;23(5):1033–6.
50. Husby KA, Huber MJ, Phillips I, et al. Vestibulovaginal leiomyosarcoma in a mare. Equine Vet Educ 2019;31(3):126–9.
51. Valentine BA. Equine Melanocytic Tumors: A Retrospective Study of 53 Horses (1988 to 1991). Veterinary Internal Medicne 1995;9(5):291–7.
52. Kumbhani TR, Raval SH, Parmar RS, et al. Vulvar Complex Apocrine Carcinoma in a Horse (Equus caballus): A Case Report and Review of Literature. J Equine Vet Sci 2023;127:104495.
53. Smith MA, Levine DG, Getman LM, et al. Vulvar squamous cell carcinoma in situ within viral papillomas in an aged Quarter Horse mare. Equine Vet Educ 2009;21(1):11–6.
54. Hedau M, Ingole RS, Sonwane S, et al. Vulvar squamous cell carcinoma in a horse: a case report. IJSRM 2017;5(1):5086–8.
55. Brandstetter LR, Doyle-Jones PS, McKenzie HC. Persistent vaginal haemorrhage due to a uterine leiomyoma in a mare. Equine Vet Educ 2010;17(3):156–8.
56. Berezowski C. Diagnosis of a uterine leiomyoma using hysteroscopy and a partial ovariohysterectomy in a mare. Can Vet J 2002;43(12):968.
57. Lopez C, Ciccarelli M, Gold JR, et al. Uterine adenocarcinoma in Quarter Horse mare. Equine Vet Educ 2018;30(12):640–4.
58. Romagnoli SE, Momont HW, Hilbert BJ, et al. Multiple recurring uterocervical leiomyomas in two half-sibling Appaloosa fillies. J Am Vet Med Assoc 1987;191(11):1449–50.
59. Janicek JC, Rodgerson DH, Boone BL. Use of a hand-assisted laparoscopic technique for removal of a uterine leiomyoma in a standing mare. JAVMA (J Am Vet Med Assoc) 2004;225(6):911–4.

60. Quinn GC, Woodford NS. Infertility due to a uterine leiomyoma in a Thoroughbred mare: clinical findings, treatment and outcome. Equine Vet Educ 2010;17(3):150–5.
61. Santschi EM, Slone DE. Successful pregnancy after partial hysterectomy in two mares. J Am Vet Med Assoc 1994;205(8):1180–2.
62. Rötting AK, Freeman DE, Doyle AJ, et al. Total and partial ovariohysterectomy in seven mares. Equine Vet J 2010;36(1):29–33.
63. Santschi EM, Adams SB, Robertson JT, et al. Ovariohysterectomy in Six Mares. Vet Surg 1995;24(2):165–71.
64. Kadic DTN, Bonilla AG. A two-step ovariohysterectomy with unilateral left flank laparoscopic assistance in a Quarter Horse mare. Equine Vet Educ 2020; 32(10). https://doi.org/10.1111/eve.13131.
65. Delling U, Howard RD, Pleasant RS, et al. Hand-Assisted Laparoscopic Ovario-hysterectomy in the Mare. Vet Surg 2004;33(5):487–94.
66. McCue PM, Roser JF, Munro CJ, et al. Granulosa cell tumors of the equine ovary. Vet Clin Equine Pract 2006;22(3):799–817.
67. Sherlock CE, Lott-Ellis K, Bergren A, et al. Granulosa cell tumours in the mare: A review of 52 cases. Equine Vet Educ 2016;28(2):75–82.
68. Charman RE, McKinnon AO. A granulosa-theca cell tumour in a 15-month-old Thoroughbred filly. Aust Vet J 2007;85(3):124–5.
69. Ball BA, Conley AJ, MacLaughlin DT, et al. Expression of anti-Müllerian hormone (AMH) in equine granulosa-cell tumors and in normal equine ovaries. Theriogenology 2008;70(6):968–77.
70. Colbern GT, Reagan WJ. Ovariectomy by colpotomy in mares. 1987. Available at: https://www.cabidigitallibrary.org/doi/full/10.5555/19882207005. [Accessed 29 February 2024].
71. Carson-Dunkerley SA, Hanson RR. Ovariectomy of granulosa cell tumors in mares by use of the diagonal paramedian approach: 12 cases (1989–1995). J Am Vet Med Assoc 1997;211(2):204–6.
72. Embertson RM. Ovaries and uterus. Equine Surgery 2006;855–64.
73. Lee M, Hendrickson DA. A review of equine standing laparoscopic ovariectomy. J Equine Vet Sci 2008;28(2):105–11.
74. Sinovich M, Archer DC, Kane-Smyth J, et al. Haemoperitoneum associated with bilateral granulosa cell tumours in a pregnant mare treated by standing ovariectomy. Equine Vet Educ 2022;34(12). https://doi.org/10.1111/eve.13612.

Tumors of the Respiratory Tract

Philip Ivens, MA, VetMB, Cert EM (Int Med), DipECEIM, MRCVS[a,*],
Victoria South, MA, VetMB, CertAVP (EM), DipECEIM, MRCVS[b]

KEYWORDS

- Thoracic neoplasia • Pulmonary granular cell tumor • Lymphosarcoma • Melanoma
- Mesothelioma

KEY POINTS

- Patients with respiratory tumors commonly present with vague and nonspecific signs.
- Initially, patients with respiratory tumors may be mistakenly diagnosed as equine asthma or pneumonia.
- Metastatic disease is as likely as a primary thoracic neoplasia and carries a poor prognosis.
- Surgical removal of some pulmonary granular cell tumors may alleviate clinical signs for several years.

INTRODUCTION

For the purposes of this article, the upper respiratory tract includes nostrils, nasal cavity, paranasal sinuses, nasopharynx, soft palate, guttural pouches (eustachian tube diverticulae), larynx, and trachea is covered in the article on tumors of the head and neck. The lower respiratory tract (LRT) includes all elements of the respiratory tract within the thoracic cavity. A wide variety of cell types are present within the respiratory tract, and therefore, there is a long list of possible tumors. The article considers the more commonly occurring tumors of the LRT and therefore of most clinical relevance.

PULMONARY GRANULAR CELL TUMOR

Granular cell tumors are a rare neoplasm in animals and humans but nevertheless are reported as the most common primary neoplasm of the equine thorax.[1] The origin of the tumor was debated historically, but is mesenchymal in origin, and immunohistochemical analysis suggests these tumors derive from Schwann cells of the peripheral nervous

---

[a] Buckingham Equine Vets Ltd, Sparrow Lodge Farm, Wicken Park Road, Wicken, Milton Keynes, MK19 6BZ, UK; [b] Department of Veterinary Medicine, University of Cambridge, Madingley Road, Cambridge, CB3 0ES, UK
* Corresponding author.
E-mail address: philip@buckinghamequinevets.com
Twitter: @victoria_south (V.S.)

Vet Clin Equine 40 (2024) 501–512
https://doi.org/10.1016/j.cveq.2024.07.013   vetequine.theclinics.com
0749-0739/24/© 2024 Elsevier Inc. All rights reserved, including those for text and data mining, AI training, and similar technologies.

system in peribronchial and peribronchiolar tissue.[2] Reports in the literature are limited to small case series, or individual case reports of individual novel aspects of the patient, management, or distribution (**Table 1**).

Granular cell tumors are locally invasive, with a nodular appearance. They may protrude into the airway lumen, eventually causing a degree of obstruction. They tend to have low metastatic potential, restricted to the pulmonary tissue.[1,3] One case series review highlighted that mares are overrepresented, but there was no age or breed predisposition.[3]

Common clinical signs in affected horses include chronic coughing, increased respiratory rate, and exercise intolerance (from airway dysfunction or the coughing itself). Horses with this tumor may be erroneously diagnosed with equine asthma, due to the similarity in initial presentation. It may be that a lack of response to routine asthma medication results in a case review, whereby the diagnosis of a granular cell tumor is revealed. If left undiagnosed, eventually the space-occupying nature of the tumor's growth leads to signs of overt respiratory obstruction such as tachypnea, increased respiratory effort, and absent or adventitious lung sounds.

Reported non-respiratory signs include weight loss, depression, anorexia, and pyrexia. Notably, the unusual medical phenomenon known as hypertrophic osteopathy (HO) has been reported with this condition (**Box 1**).[4] HO causes limb swellings that are usually bilaterally (or quadrilaterally) symmetric.

Thoracic radiography and lower airway endoscopy are logical next steps in patients presenting with this characteristically vague respiratory presentation. In cases of granular cell neoplasia, radiographs reveal well-defined single or multifocal nodules associated with the main bronchus or more widely distributed in the lung parenchyma. If there is focal secondary bacterial pneumonia present around the tumor, the radiographic appearance may include an irregular bronchoalveolar pattern that may indeed obscure the nodular shape of the primary mass. An interstitial pulmonary pattern in the ventral lung distinct from the neoplastic nodules has also been reported.[4]

The endoscopy appearance of granular cell tumors is a smooth, pink to white surfaced mass that is partly occluding a large caliber airway. It is often a mainstem bronchus that is affected. Biopsy via the endoscope may be attempted but a false negative result may be obtained with small mucosal pinch biopsies since the epithelium overlying the neoplasm will likely be normal.[3] To obtain a large tissue biopsy, a tracheostomy at the thoracic inlet may be performed to enable larger instruments (such as uterine biopsy forceps) access to the tumor site.[5]

Granular cell tumors are reportedly slow growing and have been described as incidental findings at postmortem in some horses. Conservative treatment may be appropriate, in horses with subtle and stable signs. Triggers for more intensive intervention are the secondary consequences of the tumor's presence such as focal pneumonia, coughing from airway hypersensitivity, respiratory dysfunction due to the size of the mass, or the extent of multiple masses. Removal of the intra-luminal portion of the mass via endoscopic guidance may be sufficient to alleviate clinical signs. Entire lung lobe resection has also been reported. Long-term follow-up is not reported in many cases, but where it has, horses were free from signs, with no visible tumor recurrence up to 2 years later.[6]

LYMPHOMA

Lymphoma is the most common thoracic neoplasm in horses, comprising 38% to 54% of cases.[7,8] Lymphoma involving the mediastinum is the commonest type of thoracic neoplasia identified in the horse.[9] Cases present in either mediastinal, alimentary,

Table 1

Summary of clinical signs of pulmonary neoplasms and their reported cases

	Neoplasm	Presentation	Clinical Features	Reported Cases
1° Neoplasm	Granular cell tumor	Chronic cough Tachypnoea Exercise intolerance. Weight loss, depression, and pyrexia	Hypertrophic osteopathy Single/multifocal nodules within the main bronchus/parenchyma are seen on radiographs and endoscopy.	Davis & Rush,[1] 2013 Kagawa et al,[2] 2001 Pusterla et al,[3] 2003 Heinola et al,[4] 2001 Facemire et al,[5] 2000 Ohnesorge et al,[6] 2002
2° Neoplasm	Lymphoma	Inappetence, weight loss, tachypnoea/ dyspnoea. Ventral thoracic and pectoral edema. Jugular venous distension, pulsation, and dysphagia. Mass protruding from thoracic inlet	Hypoalbuminaemia Pleural effusion on auscultation and ultrasound. Modified transudate/ non-septic exudate. Hypercalcemia (ionized) may be seen in up to 25% of cases.	Mair & Brown,[9] 1985 Mair & Hillyer,[10] 1992 Mair et al,[11] 2004 Garber et al,[12] 1994 Peroni et al,[13] 2001 Peroni et al,[14] 2000 Pollock & Russell,[15] 2006 Vachon & Fisher,[16] 1998
	Melanoma	Inappetence, weight loss Tachypnoea/dyspnoea	Pleural effusion on auscultation and ultrasound.	Valentine,[18] 1995 Milne,[21] 1986 Murray et al,[22] 1997
	Mesothelioma	Tachypnoea/dyspnoea Depression, pleural pain.	Pleural effusion on auscultation and ultrasound. Multiple soft tissue irregular cauliflower-like or plaque-like masses adherent to the pleura	Colbourne et al,[23] 1992 Kramer et al,[24] 1976 Fry et al,[25] 2003 Stoica et al,[27] 2004 Fortin et al,[28] 2018 Passantino et al,[29] 2022

> **Box 1**
> **Clinical features and diagnostic imaging findings in hypertrophic osteopathy (Marie's disease)[8]**
>
> - Classically reported in horses with an intrathoracic mass, although sometimes occurs with non-thoracic lesions.
> - Associated with neoplasia, but also reported with infection and trauma in the thoracic cavity.
> - Intrathoracic neoplastic conditions associated with HO include squamous cell carcinoma (SCC), granular cell tumor, and pulmonary metastasis.
> - Intrathoracic nonneoplastic conditions associated with HO include cranial mediastinal abscessation, pulmonary granuloma, pulmonary infarction, pleuropneumonia, and rib fracture with adhesion formation.
> - Best considered as a rare syndrome infrequently triggered by a rare primary or secondary thoracic condition.
> - The detection of HO in a patient should alert the attending veterinarian to the potential for intrathoracic disease (although non-thoracic conditions can also trigger HO).
> - Horses with HO present with bilaterally symmetric limb edema, which may be cool and comfortable or may have heat and pain upon palpation.
> - Understandably, patients with HO show stiffness and nonspecific signs of pain.
> - Radiographic findings associated with HO include palisading periosteal new bone formation perpendicular to the cortex, along the diaphyses and metaphyses of appendicular bones.
> - Anecdotally, HO has also been reported to manifest in the mandible, maxilla, and nasal bones.
> - HO may resolve if the primary condition is successfully treated.

cutaneous, or generalized forms or combinations thereof but sit under the umbrella of multicentric lymphoma.

Clinical signs are often nonspecific including inappetence and weight loss. Additionally, mediastinal lymphoma patients may develop a large volume pleural effusion that induces tachypnoea and dyspnoea. Hypoalbuminemia (loss from concurrent enteropathy or into the effusion) leads to ventral thoracic and pectoral edema. Hypercalcemia of malignancy is the most common paraneoplastic syndrome in horses and may be anticipated in up to 25% of lymphoma cases. This should be checked for via measurement of plasma ionized calcium, since *total* calcium concentrations could be artifactually within reference intervals if there is concurrent hypoalbuminemia. Cases generally have a very rapid course with a mean duration of clinical signs prior to euthanasia of approximately 4 weeks.[10] Auscultation of the chest may suggest a pleural effusion (muffled lung sounds in the ventral thorax and cardiac sounds dispersed over a larger than normal area). Intrathoracic organs and great vessels may become compressed due to the physical size of the neoplasm(s) leading to jugular venous distension and pulsation, and dysphagia.[11]

Diagnosis of thoracic lymphoma is based on clinical signs, identification of a pleural effusion, pleural fluid cytology, and biopsy of any accessible mass(es). A mass may protrude out of the thoracic inlet and may be accessible enough for surgical biopsy. Generalized peripheral lymphadenopathy is unusual. If not protruding, the neoplasm can usually be imaged ultrasonographically[12] and effusion can be sampled (**Box 2**). Pleural effusions are usually modified transudates or non-septic exudates, and neoplastic cells are frequently present in fluid; however, the absence of neoplastic cells does not rule out lymphosarcoma (false negatives are possible). Thoracoscopy can be useful to examine

Box 2
Thoracocentesis—top tips

- Locate a suitable site for thoracocentesis with ultrasound (linear or curvilinear probe).
- Blind sampling can be attempted, but is not recommended, and is hard to justify in an age of widely accessible portable ultrasound equipment.
- The cranial border of the rib should be approached, to avoid the intercostal vessels and nerves located caudal to each rib.
- Sedate the horse, then clip, and prepare the site in a sterile manner.
- Inject 5 to 10 mL local anesthetic into the skin and subcutis, perpendicular to the skin (usually a 23G, 3 cm needle).
- Make a stab incision through the skin with a number 15 scalpel blade.
- Connect an extension set and 3 way tap to the teat cannula (or spinal needle) before insertion—this reduces the risk of pneumothorax substantially.
- Be aware that puncture of the pleural can evoke a marked reaction in the horse if not adequately sedated and desensitized. Before embarking on the next step, ensure the horse is well sedated and the local site is anesthetized.
- Push the cannula through the intercostal muscles and parietal pleura into the thoracic cavity using mild, controlled pressure; when into the pleural space, a release of pressure is felt.
- Aspirate pleural fluid via syringe in a sterile manner.
- Consider appropriate analgesia during and after the procedure.

the pleural cavity and cranial mediastinum and biopsies can be taken during this procedure.[13–16]

MELANOMA

Equine melanoma is one of the most common neoplasms encountered in equine veterinary practice. They affect mainly aged, gray, horses, occasionally nonpigmented horses (white/albino or cremello) and rarely horses of another color.[17] Equine melanocytic tumors are formally categorized into 4 groups: (1) melanocytic nevi, (2) the malignant anaplastic melanoma, (3) discrete dermal melanoma, and (4) dermal melanomatosis.[18] Most melanomas appear slow growing, usually heavily pigmented (black), firm, solitary or multiple discrete to coalescing subcutaneous, and locally invasive masses. A polygenetic basis is proposed for dermal melanoma.[19,20]

Thoracic melanoma appears to be unusual.[7] There are a couple of reports of intrathoracic melanoma that had signs of sympathetic denervation[21,22] resulting in cutaneous hyperthermia with and without signs of Horner's syndrome (including sweating, ptosis, miosis, and enophthalmos) depending on the neuroanatomic location of the offending mass. In more general melanomatosis, lesions can be found throughout the thoracic cavity. Horses often present with vague inappetence and weight loss, with localizing signs of tachypnoea and dyspnoea because of pulmonary consolidation/atelectasis and voluminous pleural effusion.

CASE STUDY
History

A 19 year old, gray Connemara gelding initially presented with inappetence and pyrexia (39.6°C) and received intravenous flunixin meglumine (1.1 mg/kg bid) and oral potentiated sulfonamides (30 mg/kg bid). After 3 days, the horse developed dyspnoea and tachypnoea, and so dexamethasone (0.1 mg/kg sid IV) was administered, alongside inhaled beclomethasone (1500 μg bid) and a change of antimicrobials (to cefquinome). A week after the initial presentation, the horse underwent a respiratory endoscopy that revealed a collapsing trachea and grade 1 out of 4 mucopus. A tracheal aspirate was collected at this time. Given the persistence of respiratory signs despite antimicrobials and glucocorticoids, further diagnostics were performed including thoracic radiography and ultrasound.

Clinical Examination

Upon arrival at the referral center (8 days after the start of clinical signs), the horse was depressed but alert to stimuli. Signs of cardiorespiratory dysfunction were present including cyanotic mucous membranes, and a jugular pulse visible to the mid-cervical region. A moderate tachycardia (60 beats per minute) was present and muffled cardiac sounds were noted upon auscultation. Tachypnoea was present (28 breaths per minute) with inspiratory wheezes audible dorsally. There was a marked abdominal 2 phase effort to the breathing pattern. From the mid-thorax ventrally, bronchovesicular sounds were decreased compared to the level of respiratory effort. On percussion, there was dullness in the ventral thorax. The patient reacted to thoracic percussion that was suggestive of pleurodynia, and the horse was reluctant to move. Temperature was 39.7°C despite nonsteroidal anti-inflammatory drug administration. Borborygmi was present in all 4 abdominal quadrants.

Thoracic Ultrasound

A marked bilateral pleural effusion was imaged up to 10 cm above the point of the shoulder. The fluid was hypoechoic in nature. There was clear evidence of lung atelectasis (where the pulmonary parenchyma is compressed by the pressure of the effusion). No primary lesions within the pulmonary parenchyma were detected, except moderate "comet-tailing" of the visceral pleural surface. There were multiple round to irregular nodule-like structures attached to the diaphragm, visceral, and parietal pleural surfaces and extending into the pleural fluid, which were more hypoechoic than the juxtaposed atelectic lung. The pericardiodiaphragmatic ligament was visualized distinctly to these nodules.

Thoracocentesis

Thirty liters of a straw-colored fluid was removed through a 12G thoracic cannula. The horse's respiratory pattern improved markedly as the fluid was removed (**Fig. 1**).

Laboratory Analysis

Pleural fluid
Total nucleated cell count (TNCC)—0.50 10^9/L.
    Total protein: 23.3 g/L.

Cytology
Clear, straw-colored pleural fluid-containing few particles. Direct smears had very low nucleated cellularity; however, squash preparation of the particles revealed large clots trapping many nucleated cells (thus measured TNCC is falsely decreased). Low numbers of erythrocytes and low numbers of lysed cells are present.

Cytocentrifuge preparation also had a low cellularity. A 100 cell differential count showed.

- 75% macrophages (frequently vacuolated, many hemosiderophages, multiple melanomacrophages, rare leukophages),

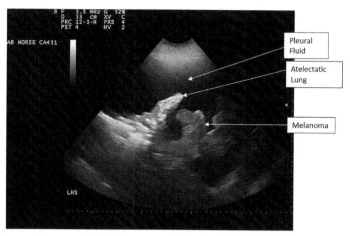

Fig. 1. Ultrasound image of the left thorax at the level of the point of the shoulder; intercostal space 7 taken with a curvilinear 2 to 5 mHz probe.

- 16% non-degenerative neutrophils, and
- 9% lymphocytes (predominantly small, mature, and rarely medium sized) and occasional reactive mesothelial cells (occasionally binucleated and occasionally with 1–3 prominent nucleoli).

The large clots in the squash preparation contain frequent melanin-containing cells, mostly being melanomacrophages, however, occasional spindle-shaped cells also seen with fine individual granules.

The background contained low numbers of melanin granules. No microorganisms were seen.

Cytology summary: Evidence of suspected neoplastic melanoma infiltration into the thoracic cavity.

Culture
No microorganisms grown.

Clinical Progression

As is often the case, the patient improved in demeanor, respiratory function, and appetite after the thoracocentesis and thoracic drainage. However, signs deteriorated the following day and in light of the pleural fluid cytologic findings; a presumptive diagnosis of intrathoracic malignant melanoma was made. The owner elected to euthanase the patient.

POSTMORTEM

Postmortem confirmed the presence of multiple black nodule-like masses within the thoracic cavity consistent with malignant melanoma/melanomatosis; similar masses were detected multifocally throughout the abdominal cavity including the spleen and liver (**Figs. 2–4**).

MESOTHELIOMA

Mesothelioma is a rare malignant mesodermal neoplasm arising from the mesothelial cells that normally form a lining one cell thick covering the peritoneal, pericardial, and pleural surfaces.[17]

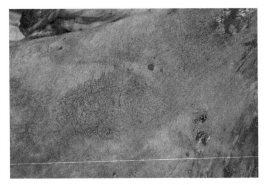

Fig. 2. Postmortem: black nodule-like masses in the pulmonary tissue in a 19 year old gray gelding with respiratory signs and pyrexia.

Mesotheliomas have been classified into 3 main histologic types:

1. Epithelioid
2. Biphasic
3. Sarcomatoid

Mesothelioma of the pleural surfaces presents with respiratory distress, depression, and pleural pain.[23] These signs typically arise from the marked thoracic effusion.[24] Ultrasound examination is often very helpful in characterizing the effusion and reveals multiple soft tissue irregular cauliflower-like masses adherent to the pleura of mixed echogenicity. Cytology of pleural fluid can be diagnostic[24] but can be difficult. Ultrasound-guided trucut biopsy and/or thoracoscopy[25] can guide diagnosis if cytology is not conclusive. Histopathological examination of mesotheliomas can be challenging to distinguish from nonneoplastic reactive mesothelial cells and other neoplasms.[26] Immunohistochemistry can help in the diagnosis of mesothelioma including calretinin.[27] Concurrent neoplasms have been documented with mesotheliomas including thyroid C-cell adenoma.[28] Bilateral body cavity mesotheliomas can also occur resulting in clinical signs from the abdominal cavity as well as the thoracic cavity.[29–31] In these patients, the most remarkable feature is the magnitude of the abdominal distension—they are often so wide that they do not fit into restraining stocks when compared to other patients of a similar height. No treatment is currently available and

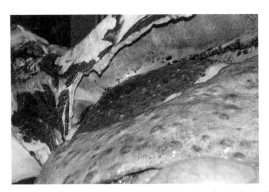

Fig. 3. Postmortem: multifocal black nodule-like masses in the spleen, liver, and parietal peritoneum of a 19 year old gray gelding with respiratory signs and pyrexia.

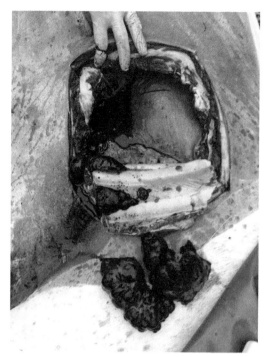

Fig. 4. Postmortem: a large multilobulated black nodule-like mass cranial mediastinum of a 19 year old gray gelding with respiratory signs and pyrexia.

clinical progression is rapid and most cases result in death or euthanasia on welfare grounds within a matter of days to weeks.

OTHER PRIMARY THORACIC NEOPLASIA

Other primary thoracic tumors are reported in the literature but appear to be relatively rare in the horse[1] and they invariably appear in the literature as individual case reports. There is an reported case of a primary bronchogenic SCC in the thorax but it seems to be a very rare location for SCC. Other tumors include thymic neoplasia, adenocarcinoma, bronchial myxoma, pleuropulmonary blastoma, pulmonary chondrosarcoma, and pulmonary leiomyosarcoma. Commonly horses with these tumors initially show vague signs of illness and weight loss. Low-grade respiratory dysfunction (from the space-occupying lesion itself or accompanying pleural effusion) may be present as the disease progresses. Consequently, just like pulmonary granular cell tumors, these rare thoracic neoplasms may be mistakenly treated as presumptive equine asthma cases initially, until the lack of response to therapy triggers a more thorough diagnostic investigation.

TUMOR-LIKE LESIONS IN THE THORAX

An important nonneoplastic differential diagnosis for thoracic neoplasia in the mature horse is equine multinodular pulmonary fibrosis (EMPF). Characteristically, this is a severe, progressive, fibrosing form of interstitial lung disease in the horse.[32] An association with equine herpes virus 5 (EHV-5) is reported in the literature, but direct evidence of causation is lacking and challenging since EHV-5 is ubiquitous in the equine population.

Box 3
Percutaneous lung biopsy—top tips

- Locate a suitable site for lung biopsy with ultrasound (linear or curvilinear probe)—locating an area with consolidation/nodular/mass where color flow Doppler can be applied to check for prominent vasculature. This diminishes the risk of significant, life-threatening, or fatal hemorrhage associated with lung biopsy, but owners must still be well informed regarding the riskiness of this procedure.
- Blind sampling is not easily justifiable in an age of widely accessible portable ultrasound equipment.
- As with thoracocentesis, the cranial border of the rib should be approached, to avoid the intercostal vessels and nerves located caudal to each rib.
- Sedate the horse, then clip, and prepare the site in a sterile manner. Consider butorphanol or morphine as part of the sedation protocol to reduce coughing during and after the procedure.
- Inject 5 to 10 mL local anesthetic into the skin and subcutis, perpendicular to the skin (usually a 23G, 3 cm needle).
- Make a stab incision through the skin with a number 15 scalpel blade.
- Either a standard trucut needle (14G or 16G) can be used to obtain lung biopsies, but an automated firing device is preferable for this procedure because it preserves the lung parenchyma better than hand-fired devices (reduces fragmentation), and the procedure can be completed more rapidly and reliably (no false firing).
- Complications are anticipated in approximately 10% of patients, and signs include coughing, hemoptysis, epistaxis, tachypnoea, and signs of pain.
- It may be appropriate to administer periprocedural tranexamic acid to support hemostasis, depending on the context of the case.

Typical clinical signs include intermittent fever, weight loss, depression, inappetence, tachypnoea, respiratory dysfunction, and coughing; clearly a similar clinical manifestation to the tumors described earlier.

Radiographically, EMPF lesions affect the interstitium and may be nodular or miliary, or both, and there can be a secondary opportunistic bacterial pneumonia.[33] A pleural effusion is less likely with EMPF than in thoracic neoplasia, unless there is a substantial concurrent bacterial pneumonia. The opportunity to biopsy nodular masses may be taken if there are superficial nodules apparent upon transthoracic ultrasound examination.[33,34] Treatment of EMPF includes valacyclovir and corticosteroids and there are reports of complete clinical resolution in the literature. There may be a better prognosis for EMPF relative to most cases of intrathoracic neoplasia (excluding some surgical candidates with granular cell tumor). Thus, where cases present with pulmonary consolidation and nodular masses, there is a strong argument for collection of percutaneous lung biopsies where possible, to differentiate these conditions (**Box 3**).

DISCLOSURE

The authors have nothing to disclose.

REFERENCES

1. Davis EG, Rush BR. Diagnostic challenges: Equine thoracic neoplasia. Equine Vet Educ 2013;25:96–107.

2. Kagawa Y, Hirayama K, Tagami M, et al. Immunohistochemical Analysis of Equine Pulmonary Granular Cell Tumours. J Comp Pathol 2001;124:122–7.
3. Pusterla N, Norris AJ, Stacy BA, et al. Granular cell tumours in the lungs of three horses. Vet Rec 2003;153:530.
4. Heinola T, Heikkilä M, Sukura A, et al. Hypertrophic pulmonary osteopathy associated with granular cell tumour in a mare. Vet Rec 2001;149:307–8.
5. Facemire PR, Chilcoat CD, Sojka JE, et al. Treatment of granular cell tumor via complete right lung resection in a horse. J Am Vet Med Assoc 2000;217:1522–5.
6. Ohnesorge B, Gehlen H, Wohlsein P. Transendoscopic Electrosurgery of an Equine Pulmonary Granular Cell Tumor. Vet Surg 2002;31:375–8.
7. Mair TS, Brown PJ. Clinical and pathological features of thoracic neoplasia in the horse. Equine Vet J 1993;25:220–3.
8. Sweeney CR, Gillette DM. Thoracic neoplasia in equids: 35 cases (1967-1987). J Am Vet Med Assoc 1989;195:374–7.
9. Mair TS, Lane JG, Lucke VM. Clinicopathological features of lymphosarcoma involving the thoracic cavity in the horse. Equine Vet J 1985;17:428–33.
10. Mair TS, Hillyer MH. Clinical features of lymphosarcoma in the horse: 77 cases. Equine Vet Educ 1992;4:108–13.
11. Mair TS, Rush BR, Tucker RL. Clinical and diagnostic features of thoracic neoplasia in the horse. Equine Vet Educ 2004;16:30–6.
12. Garber JL, Reef VB, Reimer JM. Sonographic findings in horses with mediastinal lymphosarcoma: 13 cases (1985-1992). J Am Vet Med Assoc 1994;205:1432–6.
13. Peroni JF, Horner NT, Robinson NE, et al. Equine thoracoscopy: normal anatomy and surgical technique. Equine Vet J 2001;33:231–7.
14. Peroni JF, Robinson NE, Stick JA, et al. Pleuropulmonary and cardiovascular consequences of thoracoscopy performed in healthy standing horses. Equine Vet J 2000;32:280–6.
15. Pollock PJ, Russell T. Standing thoracoscopy in the diagnosis of lymphosarcoma in a horse. Vet Rec 2006;159:354.
16. VACHON AM, Fischer AT. Thoracoscopy in the horse: diagnostic and therapeutic indications in 28 cases. Equine Vet J 1998;30:467–75.
17. Knottenbelt DC, Patterson-Kane JC, Snalune KL. Clinical Equine Oncology. Sect. III: Pr.'s Guid. equine tumours 2015;474–511. https://doi.org/10.1016/b978-0-7020-4266-9.00029-5.
18. Valentine BA. Equine Melanocytic Tumors: A Retrospective Study of 53 Horses (1988 to 1991). J Vet Intern Med 1995;9:291–7.
19. Pielberg GR, Golovko A, Sundström E, et al. A cis-acting regulatory mutation causes premature hair graying and susceptibility to melanoma in the horse. Nat Genet 2008;40:1004–9.
20. Druml T, Brem G, Horna M, et al. A Putative Candidate Gene For Melanoma Etiopathogenesis in Gray Horses. J Equine Vet Sci 2022;108:103797.
21. MILNE JC. Malignant melanomas causing Horner's syndrome in a horse. Equine Vet J 1986;18:74–5.
22. Murray MJ, Cavey DM, Feldman BF, et al. Signs of Sympathetic Denervation Associated With a Thoracic Melanoma in a Horse. J Vet Intern Med 1997;11:199–203.
23. Colbourne C, Bolton JR, Mills JN, et al. Mesothelioma in horses. Aust Vet J 1992;69:275–8.
24. Kramer JW, Nickels FA, Bell T. Cytology of Diffuse Mesothelioma in the Thorax of a Horse. Equine Vet J 1976;8:81–3.
25. Fry MM, Magdesian KG, Judy CE, et al. Antemortem diagnosis of equine mesothelioma by pleural biopsy. Equine Vet J 2003;35:723–7.

26. Husain AN, Colby TV, Ordóñez NG, et al. Guidelines for Pathologic Diagnosis of Malignant Mesothelioma: 2017 Update of the Consensus Statement From the International Mesothelioma Interest Group. Arch Pathol Lab Med 2017;142:89–108.

27. Stoica G, Cohen N, Mendes O, et al. Use of Immunohistochemical Marker Calretinin in the Diagnosis of a Diffuse Malignant Metastatic Mesothelioma in an Equine. J Vet Diagn Invest 2004;16:240–3.

28. Fortin JS, Royal AB, Kuroki K. Concurrent thoracic mesothelioma and thyroid C-cell adenoma with amyloid deposition in an aged horse. Vet Med Sci 2018;4:63–70.

29. Passantino G, Sassi E, Filippi I, et al. Thoracic and Abdominal Mesothelioma in an Older Horse in Lazio Region. Animals 2022;12:2560.

30. Heesewijk NV, Knowles EJ, Palgrave CJ, et al. Laser therapy of pulmonary granular cell tumour. Equine Vet Educ 2015;27:302–5.

31. SCARRATT WK, Crisman MV, Sponenberg DP, et al. Pulmonary granular cell tumour in 2 horses. Equine Vet J 1993;25:244–7.

32. Wong DM, Belgrave RL, Williams KJ, et al. Multinodular pulmonary fibrosis in five horses. J Am Vet Med Assoc 2008;232:898–905.

33. Lauteri E, Tortereau A, Peyrecave X, et al. Equine multinodular pulmonary fibrosis and presumed corticosteroid-induced side effects in a horse. Equine Vet Educ 2023;35:e563–70.

34. Easton-Jones CA, Cissell DD, Mohr FC, et al. Prognostic indicators and long-term survival in 14 horses with equine multinodular pulmonary fibrosis. Equine Vet Educ 2020;32:41–6.

Unusual Equine Tumors

Constanze Fintl, BVSc, MSc, PhD, Dipl ECEIM[a],*,
Pamela A. Wilkins, DVM, PhD, ACVIM-LA, ACVECC[b]

KEYWORDS

- Tumor • Horse • Mast cell • Muscle • Vascular • Neuroendocrine

KEY POINTS

- There are a number of unusual tumors in the horse.
- The clinical presentation varies widely depending on the tumor origin ranging from localized incidental findings to extensive tissue infiltration and metastatic spread.
- Immunohistochemical markers may be required to identify poorly differentiated tumors.
- Surgical excision, where possible, is frequently the first choice of treatment while ancillary treatment modalities are still less commonly reported.
- Prognosis depends on the type and size of the tumor, its location, and metastatic spread.

MAST CELL TUMORS

Mast cell tumors (MCT) are uncommon equine cutaneous tumors. The vast majority are benign and carry a good prognosis, although some cause problems because of their anatomic location. In contrast, MCT are commonly reported in other species, and are often locally aggressive and with metastatic potential.[1]

While skin tumors are the most commonly reported neoplasia in the horse, MCT prevalence ranges from 3.4% to 7.0%, with Arabian and male horses possibly over-represented.[2-5] The age group is wide, ranging from 1 to 30 years, although young adult horses are most frequently described.[2-4]

MCT are usually solitary, although they may be multiple, firm non-painful nodules within the dermis, subcutis, or superficial musculature varying in size from 0.5 to 20 cm diameter.[2,4-6] The skin may be intact or ulcerated with caseous, necrotic material occasionally discharging from the mass.[2,5] Hyperpigmentation and alopecia, with and without pruritis, have also been reported.[5]

[a] Department of Companion Animal Clinical Sciences, Faculty of Veterinary Medicine and Biosciences, Norwegian University of Life Sciences, Ås, Norway; [b] Department of Veterinary Clinical Medicine, College of Veterinary Medicine, University of Illinois at Urbana-Champaign, Urbana, IL 61802, USA
* Corresponding author. Equine Section, Department of Companion Animal Clinical Sciences, Faculty of Veterinary Medicine, Norwegian University of Life Sciences, PO Box 5003, Ås N-1432, Norway.
E-mail address: Constanze.Fintl@nmbu.no

Vet Clin Equine 40 (2024) 513–524
https://doi.org/10.1016/j.cveq.2024.07.014   **vetequine.theclinics.com**
0749-0739/24/© 2024 Elsevier Inc. All rights reserved, including those for text and data mining, AI training, and similar technologies.

MCT are most frequently located on the head (peri/orbital area, nostrils, and lips), followed by the neck, trunk, and limbs.[2,4,5,7] Other reported locations include the respiratory tract and testicles, while lameness or joint swelling resulting from primary interosseous and joint involvement has also been described.[2,8–12] Regardless of location, MCT typically display slow, progressive growth, although sudden, rapid growth may occur.[5]

Metastatic MCT with dissemination to regional lymph nodes, different organs and body cavities are rarely reported in horses.[13–15] Similarly, although typically seen in the adult horse, MCT has been reported in a neonate, although spontaneous regression of most lesions suggested similarities to cutaneous mastocytosis in humans.[16]

The underlying pathogenesis of MCT is not known and there is still some debate as to whether some lesions are truly neoplastic.[17] The argument against a neoplastic process is the benign clinical behavior and the typically well differentiated, mature cells with a low mitotic rate. However, the cytologic and histologic behavior and therefore classification is not well described in the horse and may vary. It therefore seems sensible to characterize MCT as accurately as possible, hence hematoxylin and eosin (H&E), toluidine blue staining, and c-Kit (CD117) immunohistochemical labeling are prudent.[18]

A presumptive diagnosis can be made based on fine needle aspirate (FNA) or impression smears of biopsy specimens, although histopathological evaluation is required for final confirmation.

Treatment is typically surgical removal, although the anatomic location may present challenges. The prognosis following removal is good even without clean surgical margins.[5]

CLINICS CARE POINTS

- MCT are uncommon in the horse, representing 3.4% to 7% of all skin tumors.
- The vast majority are benign and only rarely do they metastasize.
- Diagnosis is based on H&E and toluidine blue staining, while c-Kit (CD117) immunohistochemistry may help determine malignancy.
- Treatment is surgical removal.

RHABDOMYOMAS AND RHABDOMYOSARCOMAS

Tumors of striated muscle cells, both benign rhabdomyomas (RM) and malignant rhabdomyosarcomas (RMS), are rarely encountered in the horse.[19,20] They are thought to develop from pluripotential stem cells rather than well-differentiated skeletal muscle cells, thus they occasionally appear in anatomic sites not normally containing striated muscle.[20] It also explains the variety of cell morphologies encountered and the challenges of tumor characterization. In comparison, RMS is the most commonly reported soft tissue sarcoma in children with significant progress made in diagnosis, characterization, treatment, and prognosis.[21]

Histologic surveys and case series confirm the rarity of striated muscle tumors, with case reports most frequently describing RMS.[22–32] There does not appear to be a breed or sex predilection for either RM or RMS, and the reported age is wide, from the newborn foal to 21 years, although the majority of cases were young, similar to that described in humans.[21,24–32]

Clinical presentation depends on tumor localization, size, degree of local tissue invasiveness, and metastatic spread. RMS, the most frequently described form, has been recorded in skeletal muscle of the limbs, tongue, masseter muscle and body wall, but also in the urogenital tract (UGT) originating from pluripotential mesodermal cells of the urogenital ridge during embryogenesis.[22,24,25,27–30]

RMS and RM may have different appearances. RM have generally been described as well-circumscribed, unencapsulated, pale and sometimes fleshy masses,[19,26,32] while RMS may be well demarcated and partially or completely encapsulated, but also non-encapsulated, multilobular and with tissue infiltration.[19,25–32] Similarly, the rate of growth for both tumor types may vary, and recorded RMS size range from 1 to 25 cm in diameter.[25,27,29–31]

Biopsy and histopathological evaluation are critical for definitive diagnosis. In those cases where no external mass is evident, further diagnostic investigation is required and different imaging modalities may be useful additional tools depending on presenting signs and suspected localization.

Non-myogenic tumors may also infiltrate normal muscle tissue making it very difficult to identify normal muscle cells or to misclassify these as RM or RMS.[20] Immunohistochemical markers may include vimentin, desmin, muscle-specific actin, and myoglobin.[20,30] Different markers are frequently required as receptor expression changes depending on stage of muscle (and tumor) differentiation.

Therapeutic options largely depend on tumor localization and the ability to successfully surgically debulk or remove the tumor in its entirety.[19,20,32] It has been proposed that the chance of success improves if the tumor mass is less than 10 cm in diameter and when not of the alveolar variety.[19,32] One horse was treated with adjunctive radiotherapy and had no recurrence at 4 years post treatment.[25] Generally speaking, RM carry a good prognosis if removed surgically, while the prognosis for RMS is generally poor.

CLINICS CARE POINTS

- RM and RMS are rare tumors in the horse.
- A wide age range has been reported, although more frequently described in young adults.
- They develop from pluripotential stem cells, hence may appear in anatomic sites not normally containing striated muscle.
- Immunohistochemistry using different markers is frequently required as their expression changes depending on stage of muscle (and tumor) differentiation.
- Prognosis for RMS is generally poor, although successful surgical treatment, with or without adjunctive radiotherapy has been described.

LEIOMYOMAS AND LEIOMYOSARCOMAS

Tumors of smooth muscle are also rare in the horse. The malignant form (leiomyosarcomas, LMS) is less frequently reported than the benign type (leiomyomas, LM) although both are typically seen in the gastrointestinal tract (GIT) and UGT.

Their prevalence is difficult to accurately determine with surveys ranging from 0% to 0.9%.[10,22,33,34] Furthermore, some previously reported smooth muscle tumors were likely gastrointestinal stromal tumors (GIST) when reexamined using more recently available immunohistochemical markers including KIT (CD117).[20] Prognostically this may not differ; however, tyrosine kinase inhibitor drugs may offer a therapeutic option for GIST.[20]

There does not appear to be any breed or sex predilections although middle aged to older horses are most commonly reported.[19,20,35]

The clinical presentation of both LM and LMS is often non-specific and depends on tumor localization. An overview of these is described in **Table 1**.

The focus of an investigation clearly depends on tumor localization and the clinical signs relating to it. If in the GIT, and where weight loss is the presenting problem, a systematic work up as for any such case is necessary. However, a biopsy is required for definitive confirmation which may not be an option unless the horse presents with an acute bout of colic requiring surgery. Endoscopic evaluation may be helpful in visualizing tumor mass(es) of the UGT and respiratory tract and can help guide biopsy sampling. FNA appears to have limited value, and biopsy material from surgically removed or debulked masses provides more reliable material for histopathological assessment and diagnosis.[20] Radiography, computed tomography (CT), and ultrasonography are other valuable imaging modalities for tumor localization, but also to assess the extent and possible local infiltration of adjacent tissue. Blood samples may only reflect localized or more generalized inflammation associated with the tumor.

Surgical removal or debulking in the absence of metastasis and with limited local tissue infiltration may have a successful outcome.[38,41] Adjunctive chemotherapy was reported in one poorly differentiated LMS of the UGT but this was unsuccessful.[40]

CLINICS CARE POINTS

- Smooth muscle tumors are rare in the horse.
- They are most frequently reported as benign tumors of the GIT or UGT but may be malignant with metastatic potential.
- Diagnosis is based on typical gross, histopathological and immunohistochemical features.
- KIT (CD117) immunohistochemistry will help differentiate GIT smooth muscle tumors from GIST.
- Surgical removal of benign LM, or slow-growing LMS may have a favorable outcome.

HEMANGIOMAS AND HEMANGIOSARCOMAS

Vascular tumors have an estimated prevalence ranging from 0.02% to 3.2% in the horse,[23,33,34,50,51] with no strong breed or sex predilections.[50–54] Benign hemangiomas are typically seen in younger animals, including neonates, and may be difficult to differentiate from vascular hamartomas.[50,51,53,55–57] Proposed definitions and characteristics of these are presented in **Table 2**. In contrast, malignant hemangiosarcomas are most commonly reported in middle-aged to older animals, although not

Table 1			
Smooth muscle tumor localization and typical clinical signs			
Tumor Localization	**GIT**[36–39]	**UGT**[40–42]	**Respiratory**[43–46]	**Others**[47–49]
Clinical Signs	Inappetence, dysphagia, weight loss, acute/chronic colic, fever	Stranguria/ hematuria, vulval discharge, infertility	Dyspnea, inspiratory noise, exercise intolerance	Ataxia, lameness, ocular pain

Table 2
Proposed definitions of hemangiomas and hamartomas[50,51]

Nomenclature	Definition	Characteristics
Hemangioma	Benign vascular neoplasm	Capable of independent growth
Vascular hamartoma	Overgrowth of normal endothelium	Coordinated overgrowth of fully differentiated endothelial cells

exclusively so for either tumor type.[50–52,54,58] Exposure to ultraviolet radiation has been suggested to play a role hemangiosarcoma development.[59]

Vascular tumors may be challenging to identify, but location and appearance of the mass (**Table 3**), as well as age of the animal should give an early indication of its cellular origin. However, horses with hemangiosarcomas frequently present with other clinical findings related to tumor dissemination making diagnosis especially challenging.

Clinical pathology is typically nonspecific, while FNAs are frequently unrewarding yielding hemorrhagic fluid without neoplastic endothelial cells.[52,54] Ultrasonography and radiography may be helpful with thoracic or abdominal involvement, while CT may be particularly helpful when head or ocular structures are involved.[52,54]

Definitive diagnosis depends on histopathological evaluation of a representative sample, ideally with immunohistochemistry, including von Willebrand factor and CD31 (platelet–endothelial cell adhesion molecule) which may help identify neoplastic cells as endothelium.[59] Hemangiosarcomas can be particularly heterogenic and hence multiple biopsies may be required.[50,59]

Hemangiomas carry a good prognosis if completely surgically excised, although recurrence is likely as the tumor is not encapsulated and may track along tissue planes.[51,57] Adjunctive therapies described include laser photocoagulation and radiation therapy as well as cryotherapy following surgical excision.[61]

Due to the highly malignant characteristics of most hemangiosarcomas, therapeutic options described have largely been palliative with limited response.[52,54] However, where early treatment is possible, the prognosis may be more favorable. Successful surgical removal has been described, with or without topical or systemic chemotherapy, radiotherapy, and interstitial brachytherapy including in cases where the margins were undefined, or the tumor disseminated.[54,72,73,75]

CLINICS CARE POINTS

- Vascular tumors have an estimated prevalence of 0.02% to 3.2% in the horse.
- Hemangiomas are typically, but not exclusively, found as cutaneous or subcutaneous lesions in the extremities of young horses.
- Hemangiosarcomas are typically seen in mature to older horses and are highly malignant and frequently disseminated.
- Histopathological features of hemangiosarcomas can vary widely within a given tumor mass and hence multiple biopsies may be required in order to ensure an accurate diagnosis.
- Immunohistochemistry may be required to identify poorly differentiated tumors.
- Complete surgical removal carries a favorable prognosis for hemangiomas.
- The prognosis is generally poor for hemangiosarcomas but surgical resection, with and without ancillary therapy, may be curative in rare cases.

Table 3
Typical clinical characteristics of hemangiomas and hemangiosarcomas[7,50–57,59–75]

Tumor Type	Primary Anatomic Site	Clinical Signs	Lesion Appearance
Hemangiomas	Distal limbs Thorax GIT UGT Ocular structures Spinal cord	Incidental findings Lameness Ocular discomfort	Varying size Red to blue/black Single or multinodular Firm or 　fluctuating Verrucose or flat +/– Blood or serosanguineous discharge +/– Ulcerated and alopecic
Hemangiosarcomas	Skeletal muscle and ocular structures Sparsely haired/lightly pigmented 　skin areas	Dependent on primary site and if 　metastasized. Diffuse, generalized symptoms including 　weight loss, lethargy, tachycardia, 　tachypnea	Soft red or black, fleshy friable masses 　serosanguineous discharge

PHEOCHROMOCYTOMAS

Pheochromocytomas are rare neuroendocrine tumors of the chromaffin cells located in the adrenal medulla. Chromaffin cells are effectively postganglionic sympathetic neurons lacking dendrites and axons which release adrenaline and noradrenaline into the circulation when signaled by preganglionic sympathetic neurons.[76]

In the horse, pheochromocytomas are most frequently described as benign and may be functional or non-functional.[77,78] Malignant forms which invade the adrenal capsule or adjacent structures, or metastasize to other sites in the body, have also been reported.[77-79]

Although chromaffin cells are principally located in the adrenal medulla, they are also found in extra-adrenal sympathetic and parasympathetic ganglia and nerve endings. Neuroendocrine tumors in these anatomic areas, including of chromaffin cells, are called paragangliomas. In the horse, paragangliomas are rarely reported but have been described in ocular tumors.[80,81]

Pheochromocytomas of the adrenal medulla are rare tumors in the horse, with a combined prevalence of 0.9% in one post-mortem study, and where the tumor was only believed to be associated with clinical signs and death in 7 of the 37 cases recorded.[78] There does not appear to be any breed or sex predilections, but the majority of cases recorded have been in adult to older horses.[77,78,82,83]

The onset of clinical signs associated with functional lesions is frequently acute with increased heart and respiratory rate, focal or generalized sweating, muscle fasciculations, pain, and anxiety, which may be caused in part by both α- and ß-adrenergic stimulation.[77,78,84-87] Abdominal pain may be related to a generalized ileus, but rupture of the pheochromocytoma and subsequent hemorrhage has also been reported.[78,82,84,85,88] Less acute clinical signs include polyuria/polydipsia, weight loss, and lethargy.[77,78] Cardiac arrythmias and histopathological evidence of cardiomyopathy and concentric hypertrophy have also been reported.[77,82,84-86] Although one would expect blood pressure elevation resulting from α-adrenergic stimulation, this appears not always to be the case and may instead fluctuate, possibly with intermittent periods of marked hypertension.[82,84,85,87]

Clinicopathological findings are frequently non-specific, although marked hyperlactatemia and hyperglycemia have been described.[77,78,82,85,87] The latter is thought to result from catecholamine stimulation of lipolysis and reduced uptake of glucose into muscle cells.[82] Other clinicopathological findings may include hemoconcentration, azotemia, elevated creatine kinase, and cardiac troponin I concentrations.[77,78,82,86]

In contrast to humans, a reference range for markers of plasma and urine catecholamine metabolites free metanephrines and normetanephrines has not been firmly established in the horse.[77,85,89]

As already recognized in human patients, a multiple endocrine neoplasia syndrome has been described in horses where multiple endocrine benign or malignant neoplastic conditions result in other, and more prominent clinical symptoms which may mask those of a pheochromocytoma.[78,85,90,91]

Making a diagnosis of a functional pheochromocytoma is challenging due to the non-specific clinical presentation. Clinical signs and changes to parameters that do not entirely fit the expected clinical picture for a presumed problem may be the only initial indication. Rectal palpation may reveal a larger tumor if located on the left side, although transabdominal and/or rectal ultrasonography are more likely to detect these.[83,87]

The majority of pheochromocytomas, both functional and incidental, are discovered during post-mortem examination. The tumor is typically unilateral and single, although multiple masses as well as bilateral tumors of variable size have been described.[77,78,82,83,85,87]

Functional pheochromocytomas may secrete epinephrine, norepinephrine, or both and the cells producing either of these may be differentiated by the location of intracellular granules. Immunohistochemical labeling of different neuropeptides is an additional important diagnostic tool and different markers have been described in the horse including synaptophysin and chromogranin A.[87]

While the prognosis of functional tumors is generally considered to be poor, O'Brien and colleagues[87] described the successful surgical removal of the left adrenal gland in mare that presented with signs of colic thought to be directly related to the tumor.

Dopamine receptors are expressed in human adrenal tumors, including pheochromocytomas, and D2 receptors have inhibitory effects on norepinephrine secretion.[85,92] Dopamine agonists may therefore have a role in preventing adrenal hypersecretion, hence drugs such as pergolide may provide a treatment option.[85,92]

CLINICS CARE POINTS

- Pheochromocytomas are rare neuroendocrine tumors in the horse.
- They are usually benign, unilateral single tumors, but may be bilateral and/or multiple.
- Functional tumors result in increased secretion of epinephrine and/or norepinephrine.
- Ante mortem diagnosis is difficult as clinical signs are suggestive but unspecific for pheochromocytoma.
- Pheochromocytomas may be part of a multiendocrine neoplastic tumor syndrome.
- Prognosis is generally poor, although successful surgical removal of a unilateral pheochromocytoma has been reported.

DISCLOSURE

The authors have nothing to disclose.

REFERENCES

1. Blackwood L, Murphy S, Buracco P, et al. European consensus document on mast cell tumours in dogs and cats. Vet Comp Oncol 2012;10:e1–29.
2. McEntee MF. Equine cutaneous mastocytoma: morphology, biological behaviour and evolution of the lesion. J Comp Pathol 1991;104:171–8.
3. Valentine BA. Survey of equine cutaneous neoplasia in the Pacific Northwest. J Vet Diagn Invest 2006;18:123–6.
4. Mair TSK C. Mast cell tumours (mastocytosis) in the horse: a review of the literature and report of 11 cases. Equine Vet Educ 2008;20:177–82.
5. Scott DW, Miller WH. Neoplasms, cysts, hamartomas, and keratoses. In: Scott DW, Miller WH, editors. Equine Dermatology. 2nd edition. St.Louis, MO: WB Saunders; 2011. p. 468–516.
6. Knottenbelt DC, Patterson-Kane JC, Snalune KL. Haematopoietic (round cell) neoplasms. In: Knottenbelt DC, Patterson-Kane JC, Snalune KL, editors. Clinical Equine Oncology. St.Louis, MO: Elsevier; 2015. p. 342–62.
7. Flores AR, Azinhaga A, Pais E, et al. Equine ocular mast cell tumor: histopathological and immunohistochemical description. J Equine Sci 2017;28:149–52.

8. Ritmeester AM, Denicola DB, Blevins WE, et al. Primary intraosseous mast cell tumour of the third phalanx in a quarter horse. Equine Vet J 1997;29:151–2.
9. Taylor S, Martinelli MJ, Trostle SS, et al. Articular mastocytosis in the tarsocrural joint of a horse. Equine Vet Educ 2005;17:207–11.
10. Knowles EJ, Tremaine WH, Pearson GR, et al. A database survey of equine tumours in the United Kingdom. Equine Vet J 2016;48:280–4.
11. Meurice A, Pujol R, Albaric O, et al. Tracheal obstructive mastocytoma in a pony. Equine Vet Educ 2023;35:e248–54.
12. Brown JA, O'Brien MA, Hodder ADJ, et al. Unilateral testicular mastocytoma in a Peruvian Paso stallion. Equine Vet Educ 2008;20:172–5.
13. Williams NJ, van den Boom R. Cutaneous mastocytoma with eosinophilia and eosinophilic infiltration of the small intestine in an Arabian gelding. Vet Rec Case Rep 2020;8:e000773.
14. Tan RH, Crisman MV, Clark SP, et al. Multicentric mastocytoma in a horse. J Vet Intern Med 2007;21:340–3.
15. Combarros D, Wilhelmi-Vilarrasa I, Lacroux C, et al. Multinodular Malignant Cutaneous Mast Cell Tumor in a Horse With Generalized Pruritus and Reactive Fibrosis: A Case Report. J Equine Vet Sci 2020;87:102921.
16. Cheville NF, Prasse K, van der Maaten M, et al. Generalized Equine Cutaneous Mastocytosis. Vet Pathol 1972;9:394–407.
17. Johnson PJ. Dermatologic tumors (excluding sarcoids). Vet Clin North Am Equine Pract 1998;14:625–58.
18. Clarke L, Simon A, Ehrhart EJ, et al. Histologic characteristics and KIT staining patterns of equine cutaneous mast cell tumors. Vet Pathol 2014;51:560–2.
19. Knottenbelt DC, Patterson-Kane JC, Snalune KL. Smooth muscle and skeletal muscle neoplasms In: Knottenbelt DC, Patterson-Kane JC. In: Snalune KL, editor. Clinical Equine Oncology. St.Louis, MO: Elsevier; 2015. p. 305–11.
20. Cooper BJ, Valentine BA. Tumors of Muscle. In: Meuten DJ, editor. Tumors in domestic animals. 5th edition. NJ, USA: Wiley; 2016. p. 425–66.
21. Skapek SX, Ferrari A, Gupta AA, et al. Rhabdomyosarcoma. Nat Rev Dis Primers 2019;5:1.
22. Baker JR, Leyland A. Histological survey of tumours of the horse, with particular reference to those ofthe skin. Vet Rec 1975;96:419–22.
23. Kerr KMA, Alden CL. Equine neoplasia – a ten year survey. Proc Am Ass Vet Lab Diagnost 1974;17:183–7.
24. Pascoe RR, Summers PM. Clinical survey of tumours and tumour-like lesions in horses in south east Queensland. Equine Vet J 1981;13:235–9.
25. Castleman WL, Toplon DE, Clark CK, et al. Rhabdomyosarcoma in 8 horses. Vet Pathol 2011;48:1144–50.
26. Hamir AN. Striated muscle tumours in horses. Vet Rec 1982;111:367–8.
27. Sohrabi Haghdoost I, Zakarian B. Neoplasms of equidae in Iran. Equine Vet J 1985;17:237–9.
28. Turnquist SE, Pace LW, Keegan K, et al. Botryoid rhabdomyosarcoma of the urinary bladder in a filly. J Vet Diagn Invest 1993;5:451–3.
29. Clegg PD, Coumbe A. Alveolar rhabdomyosarcoma: an unusual cause of lameness in a pony. Equine Vet J 1993;25:547–9.
30. Hanson PD, Frisbie DD, Dubielzig RR, et al. Rhabdomyosarcoma of the tongue in a horse. J Am Vet Med Assoc 1993;202:1281–4.
31. Aupperle H, Börgel C, Raila G, et al. Morphological, immunohistochemical, and ultrastructural findings in an embryonal rhabdomyosarcoma of a newborn Thoroughbred foal. J Equine Vet Sci 2004;24:159–64.

32. Meyerholz DK, Caston SS, Haynes JS. Congenital fetal rhabdomyoma in a foal. Vet Pathol 2004;41:518–20.
33. Bastianello SS. A survey on neoplasia in domestic species over a 40-year period from 1935 to 1974 in the Republic of South Africa. IV. Tumours occurring in Equidae. Onderstepoort J Vet Res 1983;50:91–6.
34. Sundberg JP, Burnstein T, Page EH, et al. Neoplasms of Equidae. J Am Vet Med Assoc 1977;170:150–2.
35. Knottenbelt DC, Patterson-Kane JC, Snalune KL. Tumours of the musculoskeletal system. In: Knottenbelt DC, Patterson-Kane JC, Snalune KL, editors. Clinical Equine Oncology. St.Louis, MO: Elsevier; 2015. p. 664–79.
36. Taylor SD, Pusterla N, Vaughan B, et al. Intestinal neoplasia in horses. J Vet Intern Med 2006;20:1429–36.
37. Taylor SD, Haldorson GJ, Vaughan B, et al. Gastric neoplasia in horses. J Vet Intern Med 2009;23:1097–102.
38. Miles S, Davis W, Craft W. Intramural jejunal leiomyoma as a cause of colic. Equine Vet Educ 2021;33:e104–7.
39. Faulkner J, Vlaminck L, Geerinckx L, et al. Leiomyoma of the proximal cervical oesophagus in a horse. Equine Vet Educ 2023;35:e154–9.
40. Hurcombe SD, Slovis NM, Kohn CW, et al. Poorly differentiated leiomyosarcoma of the urogenital tract in a horse. J Am Vet Med Assoc 2008;233:1908–12.
41. Husby K, Huber M, Phillips I, et al. Vestibulovaginal leiomyosarcoma in a mare. Equine Vet Educ 2019;31:126–9.
42. MacGillivray KC, Graham TD, Parente EJ. Multicentric leiomyosarcoma in a young male horse. J Am Vet Med Assoc 2003;223:1017–21.
43. Veraa S, Dijkman R, Klein W, et al. Computed tomography in the diagnosis of malignant sinonasal tumours in three horses. Equine Vet Educ 2009;21:284–8.
44. Santamaria-Martínez EA, Nevárez-Garza AM, Trejo-Chávez A, et al. Dyspnea caused by an obstructive tracheal leiomyoma in a horse: a rare case. J Equine Vet Sci 2014;34:1338–41.
45. Drew S, Meehan L, Reardon R, et al. Guttural pouch leiomyosarcoma causing nasopharyngeal compression in a pony. Equine Vet Educ 2018;30:64–9.
46. Radtke A, Caruso M, Miller A, et al. Treatment of a poorly differentiated sarcoma in the oropharynx of a horse. Equine Vet Educ 2020;32:O15–8.
47. Kawabata A, Del Piero F, Caserto BG, et al. Metastatic leiomyosarcoma causing ataxia in a horse. J Equine Vet Sci 2016;43:23–7.
48. Grosås S, Østevik L, Revold T, et al. Uveal myxoid leiomyosarcoma in a horse. Clin Case Reports 2017;5:1811.
49. Giacchi A, Marcatili M, Withers J, et al. An atypical presentation of leiomyosarcoma causing extremity compartment syndrome of the crural region in a Dutch Warmblood mare: a case report. J Vet Sci 2020;21:e3.
50. Valli V, Kiupel M, Bienzle D, et al. Hematopoietic system. In: Maxie MD, editor. Jubb, Kennedy, and Palmer's pathology of domestic animals. St. Louis, MO: Elsevier; 2016. p. 102–268.
51. Hargis AM, McElwain TF. Vascular neoplasia in the skin of horses. J Am Vet Med Assoc 1984;184:1121–4.
52. Southwood LL, Schott HC 2nd, Henry CJ, et al. Disseminated hemangiosarcoma in the horse: 35 cases. J Vet Intern Med 2000;14:105–9.
53. Metcalfe A, Craig LE. Intestinal hemangiomas in 8 horses. Vet Pathol 2024;61: 58–61.
54. Johns I, Stephen JO, Del Piero F, et al. Hemangiosarcoma in 11 young horses. J Vet Intern Med 2005;19:564–70.

55. Johnstone A. Congenital vascular tumours in the skin of horses. J Comp Pathol 1987;97:365–8.
56. Vos JH, van der Gaag I, van Dijk JE, et al. Lobular capillary haemangiomas in young horses. J Comp Pathol 1986;96:637–44.
57. Platt H. Vascular malformations and angiomatous lesions in horses: a review of 10 cases. Equine Vet J 1987;19:500–4.
58. Arenas-Gamboa AM, Mansell J. Epithelioid haemangiosarcoma in the ocular tissue of horses. J Comp Pathol 2011;144:328–33.
59. Knottenbelt DC, Patterson-Kane JC, Snalune KL. Vascular neoplasms. In: Knottenbelt DC, Patterson-Kane JC, Snalune KL, editors. Clinical Equine Oncology. St. Louis, MO: Elsevier; 2015. p. 332–41.
60. Sansom J, Donaldson D, Smith K, et al. Haemangiosarcoma involving the third eyelid in the horse: a case series. Equine Vet J 2006;38:277–82.
61. Kleiter M, Velde K, Hainisch E, et al. Radiation therapy communication: equine hemangioma. Vet Radiol Ultrasound 2009;50:560–3.
62. Jacobsen S, Christophersen M, Tnibar A, et al. Surgical treatment of a large congenital cavernous haemangioma on the thorax of a foal. Equine Vet Educ 2018;30:289–94.
63. Pool RRT, Thompson KG. Tumors of joints. In: Meuten DJ, editor. Tumors in domestic animals. 4th edition. NJ, USA: Wiley; 2002. p. 199–243.
64. Valentine BA, Ross CE, Bump JL, et al. Intramuscular hemangiosarcoma with pulmonary metastasis in a horse. J Am Vet Med Ass 1986;188:628–9.
65. Gelatt KJ, Neuwirth L, Hawkins DL, et al. Hemangioma of the distal phalanx in a colt. Vet Radiol Ultrasound 1996;37:275–80.
66. Mahne AT, Marais HJ, Rubio-Martinez LM, et al. Severe hindlimb lameness and pathological femur fracture in a horse secondary to haemangiosarcoma. Equine Vet Educ 2014;26:552–8.
67. Hughes K, Scott VHL, Blanck M, et al. Equine renal hemangiosarcoma: clinical presentation, pathologic features, and pSTAT3 expression. J Vet Diagn Invest 2018;30:268–74.
68. Ladd SM, Crisman MV, Duncan R, et al. Central nervous system hemangiosarcoma in a horse. J Vet Intern Med 2005;19:914–6.
69. Ferrucci F, Vischi A, Zucca E, et al. Multicentric hemangiosarcoma in the horse: A case report. J Equine Vet Sci 2012;32:65–71.
70. Beaumier A, Dixon C, Robinson N, et al. Primary cardiac hemangiosarcoma in a horse: echocardiographic and necropsy findings. J Vet Cardiol 2020;32:66–72.
71. Gearhart PM, Steficek BA, Peteresen-Jones SM. Hemangiosarcoma and squamous cell carcinoma in the third eyelid of a horse. Vet Ophthalmol 2007;10:121–6.
72. Scherrer NM, Lassaline M, Engiles J. Ocular and periocular hemangiosarcoma in six horses. Vet Ophthalmol 2018;21:432–7.
73. Vázquez Bringas FJ, Romero Lasheras A, Laborda García A, et al. Treatment of congenital atypical haemangiosarcoma in a foal. Equine Vet Educ 2023;35:e522–30.
74. Conturba B, Lo Feudo CM, Stucchi L, et al. Recurrent equine capillary haemangioma treated with adjunctive laser photocoagulation therapy: a case report. Vet Dermatol 2021;32:290-e78.
75. Burks B, Leonard J, Orsini J, et al. Interstitial brachytherapy in the management of haemangiosarcoma of the rostrum of the horse: case report and review of the literature. Equine Vet Educ 2009;21:487–93.
76. Rosol TJ, Meuten DJ. Tumors of the Endocrine Glands. In: Meuten DJ, editor. Tumors in domestic animals. 5th edition. NJ, USA: Wiley-Blackwell; 2016. p. 766–833.

77. Yovich J, Horney F, Hardee G. Pheochromocytoma in the horse and measurement of norepinephrine levels in horses. Can Vet J 1984;25:21.
78. Luethy D, Habecker P, Murphy B, et al. Clinical and Pathological Features of Pheochromocytoma in the Horse: A Multi-Center Retrospective Study of 37 Cases (2007-2014). J Vet Intern Med 2016;30:309–13.
79. Froscher BG, Power HT. Malignant pheochromocytoma in a foal. J Am Vet Med Assoc 1982;181:494–6.
80. Basher AW, Severin GA, Chavkin MJ, et al. Orbital neuroendocrine tumors in three horses. J Am Vet Med Assoc 1997;210:668–71.
81. Miesner T, Wilkie D, Gemensky-Metzler A, et al. Extra-adrenal paraganglioma of the equine orbit: six cases. Vet Ophthalmol 2009;12:263–8.
82. Norgate DJ, Foster A, Dunkel B, et al. Clinical features, anaesthetic management and perioperative complications seen in three horses with pheochromocytoma. Vet Rec Case Rep 2019;7:e000744.
83. Johnson PJ, Goetz TE, Foreman JH, et al. Pheochromocytoma in two horses. J Am Vet Med Assoc 1995;206:837–41.
84. Ranninger E, Bettschart-Wolfensberger R. Polymorphic tachycardia in an anaesthetised horse with an undiagnosed pheochromocytoma undergoing emergency coeliotomy. Vet Rec Case Rep 2020;8:e001000.
85. Fouché N, Gerber V, Gorgas D, et al. Catecholamine metabolism in a Shetland pony with suspected pheochromocytoma and pituitary pars intermedia dysfunction. J Vet Intern Med 2016;30:1872–8.
86. Dufourni A, De Clercq D, Vera L, et al. Pheochromocytoma in a horse with polymorphic ventricular tachycardia. Vlaams Diergeneeskundig Tijdschrift 2017;86: 241–9.
87. O'Brien TJ, Pezzanite LM, Acutt EV, et al. Successful surgical removal of a pheochromocytoma in a mare via trans-costal approach. Equine Vet J 2023;55:1012–20.
88. Yovich J, Ducharme N. Ruptured pheochromocytoma in a mare with colic. J Am Vet Med Assoc 1983;183:462–4.
89. Eisenhofer G, Goldstein DS, Walther MM, et al. Biochemical diagnosis of pheochromocytoma: how to distinguish true-from false-positive test results. J Clin Endocrin Metab 2003;88:2656–66.
90. Germann S, Rütten M, Derungs S, et al. Multiple endocrine neoplasia-like syndrome in a horse. Vet Rec Case Rep 2006;159:530–2.
91. DeCock H, MacLachlan N. Simultaneous occurrence of multiple neoplasms and hyperplasias in the adrenal and thyroid gland of the horse resembling multiple endocrine neoplasia syndrome: case report and retrospective identification of additional cases. Vet Path 1999;36:633–6.
92. Pivonello R, Ferone D, Lombardi G, et al. Novel insights in dopamine receptor physiology. Eur J Endocrinol 2007;156:S13–21.

Paraneoplastic Syndromes in Horses

Imogen Johns, BVSc, PGCAP, FRCVS,

KEYWORDS

• Cancer • Fever • Cachexia • Hypercalcemia

KEY POINTS

- A paraneoplastic syndrome (PNS) is a clinical sign or signs, or hematological/biochemical change that occurs as an indirect consequence of cancer but is NOT due to its physical presence.
- The pathogenesis remains unclear, but the symptoms are typically attributable to substances (such as hormones or cytokines) that are secreted by the tumor itself which then have distance effects throughout the body, or as a result of antibodies directed against the tumor cells that cross react with other tissues.
- Signs of a PNS may precede signs of the tumor itself by weeks to months.
- The clinical signs or hematological/biochemical changes are not pathognomonic for a specific type of tumor; as PNS are rare, these signs will typically occur with greater frequency in non-neoplastic conditions.

INTRODUCTION

A paraneoplastic syndrome (PNS) is a disease or collection of clinical signs that occur not due to the direct physical presence of a tumor (or its metastases) but as an indirect effect of the cancer.[1] In many cases, the pathogenesis of these PNS remains unclear, but the symptoms are typically attributable to substances (such as hormones or cytokines) that are secreted by the tumor itself which then have distance effects throughout the body, or as a result of antibodies directed against the tumor cells that cross react with other tissues.[1–3] While relatively rarely reported in horses, PNSs are more commonly reported in small animals[3] and humans, being seen in up to 8% of patients with cancer.[4] In many instances, the PNS signs precede the clinical signs attributable to the tumor itself and thus their recognition may allow for earlier diagnosis of the neoplastic process itself. Because earlier diagnosis can result in earlier treatment, it is possible that diagnosis of a PNS could improve outcomes in patients with neoplasia, although at present this is not routinely reported in equine medicine.

B and W Equine Hospital, Breadstone, Berkeley, Gloucestershire GL139HG, UK
E-mail address: imogen.johns@bwequinevets.co.uk

Vet Clin Equine 40 (2024) 525–535
https://doi.org/10.1016/j.cveq.2024.07.015
0749-0739/24/© 2024 Elsevier Inc. All rights reserved, including those for text and data mining, AI training, and similar technologies.

Paraneoplastic syndromes can result in a diverse range of clinical signs affecting multiple body systems.[1–3] The diagnosis of many PNSs is challenging as there are no pathognomonic signs that alert the clinician to their presence, and in many cases, the signs are more commonly associated with more "routine" diagnoses.[1,2] For example, fever is one of the more commonly reported PNS, but would far more frequently be associated with an infectious or inflammatory condition rather than neoplasia.[5,6] Similarly, pruritis is reported as a PNS, but again, would be more commonly associated with the presence of ectoparasites or immune conditions of the skin.[7,8] As such, although earlier recognition of a PNS may allow for earlier treatment of a neoplastic condition, this can be challenging due to the lack of specific clinical signs which might prompt the clinician to investigate the presence of a possible neoplastic condition.

Specific tumor types do not necessarily always induce a particular type or group of PNS signs nor can the presence of a particular PNS be used to confirm the presence of a particular type of neoplasia. For example, lymphoma in one horse may be accompanied by fever and in another horse by hypercalcemia.[1,2]

The presence of a PNS can result in significant additive morbidity separate to the physical presence of the tumor itself, and their management can complicate the treatment or management of neoplasia.[1,3,4,9] Recognition of the presence of and treatment for any PNS is thus an important part of the management of horses with neoplasia. This article will discuss the reported PNS in horses, which include cancer cachexia, fever and increased acute phase protein concentrations, hypercalcemia, and others (**Box 1**).

CACHEXIA AND ANOREXIA

Horses with advanced neoplasia typically have a poor appetite with resultant weight loss, a syndrome termed cancer related anorexia.[10,11] Cancer cachexia in contrast is weight loss and functional impairment that occurs in patients with neoplasia despite adequate nutritional intake and that cannot be reversed nutritionally.[12] Both anorexia

---

Box 1
Paraneoplastic conditions described in horses

- Anorexia and cachexia
- Fever and increased acute phase protein concentrations
- Hypercalcemia
- Hypertrophic osteopathy (Marie's disease)
- Monoclonal gammopathy
- Anemia
- Erythrocytosis
- Thrombocytopenia
- Hypoglycemia
- Amyloidosis
- Dermatologic conditions (alopecia, pruritis, bullous stomatitis)
- Hypercuprinemia

and cachexia are thought to be secondary to tumor production of catabolic cytokines such as TNF-α, IL-6, and IFN-γ.[1,9] The resultant insulin resistance and excessive fat and protein breakdown result in a severe protein-calorie malnutrition with often profound weight loss.[3,12] When present in human patients, cancer cachexia is strongly correlated with poor prognosis, a correlation which likely also exists in horses.[12] While the term cancer cachexia is rarely used in equine publications, poor body condition and weight loss are commonly listed as presenting clinical signs in horses especially with abdominal and thoracic neoplasia and as such, cancer cachexia is probably one of the more common PNS in horses.[10,11,13–17] Increasing the plane of nutrition may temporarily slow the rate of weight loss but unless the underlying cancer can be treated the condition is progressive.

FEVER AND INCREASED ACUTE PHASE PROTEIN CONCENTRATION

Fever is often reported in horses with neoplasia, and can be recurrent, undulating or persistent.[13,14,17] In 2 case series describing clinical features of intestinal neoplasia fever was recorded at presentation or historically in 9 of 34[14] and 17 of 34.[13] In a case series of 63 horses with pyrexia of unknown origin, neoplasia was identified as the cause in 14 cases, 10 of which were diagnosed with lymphoma.[5] Fever in horses with neoplasia is thought to occur either as a result of the presence of secondary infections, or by the release of endogenous pyrogens such as IL-1, IL-6, and TNF-α by the tumor itself. The latter is thought to occur more commonly in rapidly growing tumors where tissue necrosis occurs. In human patients with cancer, the majority (2 of 3) of febrile episodes are due to infection,[18] suggesting that in horses with fever and neoplasia, efforts to diagnose a secondary infection should be made rather than just assuming the fever is due to non-septic cytokine release.

Fever may be accompanied by evidence of inflammation or infection on bloodwork, such as increased concentrations of acute phase proteins (fibrinogen and serum amyloid A), increased globulin concentrations and either a leukopenia or leukocytosis.[1,2,10,13–17] Six of 24 horses with gastric squamous cell carcinoma had a leukocytosis, hyperfibrinogenemia, and hyperglobulinemia in one study[10] with a second study in horses with intestinal neoplasia identifying leukocytosis (13 of 34), hyperfibrinogenemia (11 of 34), and hyperglobulinemia (9 of 32).[14]

HYPERCALCEMIA

Hypercalcemia of malignancy (HM) is one of the more commonly reported PNS in horses[2] and can be seen in association with a number of different neoplastic processes, including squamous cell carcinoma,[10,19,20] lymphoma,[21,22] carcinomas,[22–24] ameloblastoma,[25] plasma cell myeloma,[26] multiple myeloma,[27,28] and chief cell adenoma.[29] Despite being one of the more commonly reported PNS in horses, more common causes of hypercalcemia should be considered with chronic renal failure the most common cause.[30] Other causes including iatrogenic administration of intravenous calcium, iatrogenic hypervitaminosis D ingestion of wild blooming jasmine, pseudohyperparathyroidism, and hyperparathyroidism.[2,30–33] HM is the most common cause of hypercalcemia in dogs[3] and is reported to occur in 20% of human patients with cancer, being more common in advanced disease, with its presence associated with a poorer prognosis.[34]

There are several purported causes of HM with production of parathyroid hormone-related peptide (PTHrp) by the tumor considered the most common cause.[34] Other rarer causes include ectopic parathyroid hormone (PTH) production, excessive activation of extrarenal vitamin D, and extensive bone lysis/metastasis.[34] Calcium homeostasis is regulated by calcitonin (produced by the thyroid C cells), Vitamin D (either ingested or produced by UV light) and PTH (produced by chief cells of the parathyroid gland). PTH acts to maintain calcium concentrations by increasing (1) absorption of calcium from the gastrointestinal tract in the presence of 1,25 dihydroxy vitamin D; (2) renal tubular calcium resorption; and (3) calcium reabsorption from bone, with the net result to increase serum calcium concentrations.[34] PTHrp is structurally very similar to PTH and acts on the same receptors in the bone as PTH resulting in activated osteoclasts and release of calcium into the circulation. PTHrp also acts in the renal tubules to increase calcium resorption but does not appear to increase calcium absorption from the intestine, at least in people.[34] PTHrp is produced by almost all cells in the body, but typically is present in only minute amounts. Increased concentrations have only been identified in pathologic conditions, especially malignancy where the hormone may be produced in excess amounts either by normal cells or the tumor cells themselves.[28] While an increased PTHrp concentration is the most common cause of HM in people, the frequency with which it occurs in horses is unknown as hormone levels are rarely measured. HM associated with an increased PTHrp was diagnosed in a mare with multiple myeloma although interestingly, the PTHrp concentration was initially normal despite hypercalcemia.[34] An increased PTHrp concentration (with normal PTH concentration) was evident only on re-check 7 months after the initial presentation. A locally invasive mandibular ameloblastoma resulted in HM with associated increased PTHrp. In this horse, surgical resection of the mass resolved both the increased calcium and PTHrp concentrations.[25] Extensive bone lysis either by a primary tumor or metastases appears to be relatively rare in horses and is thus considered a rare cause of HM, as is ectopic PTH production. Clinical signs associated with hypercalcemia appear to be uncommon, and in people typically only occur when calcium concentrations are markedly increased.[34] However, in theory hypercalcemia can cause muscle weakness, depression, and seizures due to elevated cerebrospinal fluid calcium concentrations.[32] Hypercalcemia can also cause a shortened Q–T interval and S–T depression with slowing of intracardiac conduction resulting in atrio-ventricular block,[35] but tachycardia may also occur.[36] In symptomatic human patients, treatments include intravenous hydration, drugs such as bisphosphonates and denosumab (a human monoclonal antibody that inhibits osteoclast formation, function, and survival) to reduce bone resorption, corticosteroids, and treatment of the underlying cause.[34] Similar protocols could be implemented in symptomatic horses to reduce calcium concentrations.

HYPERTROPHIC OSTEOPATHY

Hypertrophic osteopathy (HO; Marie's disease) is a rare condition which results in periosteal proliferation of new bone and soft tissue swelling along the diaphysis of, in particular, long bones.[37,38] The swelling appears to cause discomfort with horses presenting with swelling of the limbs and a stiff, shuffling gait. The pathogenesis is unclear, but it is predominately seen in horses with intra-thoracic disease, which may be neoplastic or non-neoplastic. In a case series and review of the literature in 42 equids with HO, intra-thoracic disease was diagnosed in 30 cases, with an inflammatory condition present in the majority.[37,38] Neoplastic conditions associated with HO include squamous cell carcinoma, granular cell myeloblastoma, both primary and metastatic lung tumors,[37,38] ovarian carcinoma,[39] gastric squamous cell carcinoma,[40] granular cell myoblastoma,[41] and pulmonary granular cell tumor.[42,43] Infectious/inflammatory conditions are reported to include nodular pulmonary fibrosis,[44] pneumonia, pulmonary abscesses, tuberculosis, pulmonary infarction, and rib fractures with chronic pleural adhesions.[37,38] No obvious cause (despite a full post mortem) was found in 4 cases,[38] and in one mare, the condition occurred in successive pregnancies.[45] Diagnosis of HO is made on the basis of characteristic clinical signs and radiographic changes showing new bone proliferation of the diaphysis. Interestingly, the bony proliferation does not affect the joints. While most commonly associated with intrathoracic disease, extra-thoracic disorders reported to cause HO in people include hepatic, cardiac, and abdominal disease.[46] With both intra and extra-thoracic neoplastic or inflammatory disorders associated with HO, it is likely that the pathogenesis is multifactorial, and currently it remains elusive. The classic pathophysiological changes in HO are increased peripheral blood flow, proliferation of vascular connective tissue, and ultimately bone spicule formation.[47,48] Most recently, it has been proposed that the release of vascular endothelial growth factor and platelet-derived growth factor from platelets and abnormal platelet circulation may be involved in HO initiation and progression.[48–53] Other proposed mechanisms include a neural reflex, increased circulating vasodilators or increased growth hormones due to decreased inactivation by the lungs or tissue hypoxia.[48,50,54,55] Treatment of HO in horses is largely unsuccessful, but has been reported following resolution of the inciting condition (treatment of intra-thoracic infection, spontaneous resolution in cases with no identified cause, removal of ovarian carcinoma).[38,39,56]

MONOCLONAL GAMMOPATHY

A monoclonal gammopathy is a PNS that can be seen in horses with myeloma-related disorders (multiple myeloma, extramedullary plasmacytoma, and solid osseous plasmacytoma) and rarely in horses with lymphoma/leukemia.[57–60] Multiple myeloma (also called plasma cell myeloma) is rarely reported in horses, with fewer than 20 cases reported in the literature.[26,28,59–72] In horses with multiple myeloma there is a neoplastic proliferation of plasma cells that primarily involves the bone marrow but may originate from extra-medullary sites[59] The neoplastic plasma cells are responsible for overproduction of a monoclonal immunoglobulin product termed paraprotein or M component. These paraproteins can consist of entire immunoglobulins, free light chains, fragments of light chains, or partial immunoglobulins (which may be missing one or both chains).[59] Routine biochemical screening will initially identify hyperproteinemia, characterized by a hyperglobulinemia and often accompanied by hypoalbuminemia.[2] Serum protein electrophoresis is used to characterize a sharply defined peak that is typically in the beta or gamma region. A polyclonal gammopathy is more commonly diagnosed and would be consistent with chronic inflammation or infection, chronic liver disease, neoplasia, and other conditions that cause nonspecific antigenic stimulation and activation of large numbers of B-cell clones, with synthesis of antibodies from all Ig types. In some horses with multiple myeloma in which the overproduced immunoglobulin is a light chain immunoglobulin, these immunoglobulins are small enough to pass through the glomerulus into the urine where they are referred to as Bence Jones proteins. Electrophoresis of urine is used to detect these proteins as they are not detected by routine dipstick analysis.[2] Monoclonal gammopathy can be occur with other PNS as evidenced by the diagnosis of hypercalcemia and high serum PTHrp in one horse with multiple myeloma.[28]

ANEMIA AND ERYTHROCYTOSIS

Anemia is commonly reported in horses with neoplasia and when characterized, is frequently normocytic normochromic suggestive of anemia of chronic inflammation.[1,2] Other causes of neoplasia-associated anemia include blood loss (in particular squamous cell carcinoma and hemangiosarcoma), premature destruction of red cells coated with antibody and immune-mediated hemolytic anemia.[10,59,73]

Erythrocytosis is defined as an absolute increase in the red cell mass and can be primary or secondary. Primary erythrocytosis occurs due to bone marrow disease, with the increased red cell mass being independent of the erythropoietin (EPO) concentration. In contrast, secondary erythropoiesis occurs as a result of increased EPO concentration due to chronic hypoxia (appropriate) or due to excessive production of EPO (inappropriate). Erythrocytosis can occur as a PNS and is typically due to tumor production of EPO or prostaglandin production by the tumor enhancing the effect of EPO.[74,75] Erythrocytosis as a PNS has been diagnosed predominately in horses with hepatic neoplasia, including hepatoblastoma and hepatocellular carcinoma[74–79] but has also been reported with metastatic carcinoma[23] and lymphoma.[80] Serum EPO concentrations are reported to be both increased and normal. Clinical signs of erythrocytosis are non-specific although most cases are reported to have markedly congested (red) mucous membranes. Treatment of PNS erythrocytosis with phlebotomy and intravenous fluids was not successful in 2 reported cases.[75,78] In one horse with suspected myosarcoma hydroxyurea was used to successfully reduce both clinical signs and packed cell volume (PCV).[1]

HYPOGLYCEMIA

Hypoglycemia is rare in adult horses with possible causes including sepsis, liver disease, gastrointestinal disease, hypertriglyceridemia, and neoplasia.[81] Paraneoplastic hypoglycemia has been described in horses with renal carcinoma, renal tubular carcinoma, renal adenocarcinoma, hemangiosarcoma, lymphoma, abdominal and pleural mesothelioma, cholangiosarcoma, and hepatocellular carcinoma.[74,79,81–86] Hypoglycemia associated with non-insulin secreting tumors in horses is believed to result from the production of insulin-like growth factor-II resulting in enhanced removal of glucose from the circulation by skeletal muscle.[83,86] Clinical signs related to the decreased blood glucose concentration can include lethargy and weakness to seizures.[81] While treatment with intravenous glucose can resolve the hypoglycemia, the prognosis is poor due to the underlying neoplasia.

OTHER PARANEOPLASTIC CONDITIONS

Other PNSs reported in humans and small animals, but rarely or not reported in horses include a syndrome of inappropriate anti-diuretic hormone secretion, neurologic and dermatologic conditions, Cushing's syndrome, thrombocytopenia, amyloidosis, and hypercuprinemia.[1,4,8,70,87–94] Whether these conditions do not occur in horses or have simply yet to be recognized is not known.

CLINICS CARE POINTS

- A paraneoplastic syndrome is a clinical sign or signs, or hematological/biochemical change that occurs as an indirect consequence of cancer but is NOT due to its physical presence.
- The pathogenesis remains unclear, but the symptoms are typically attributable to substances (such as hormones or cytokines) that are secreted by the tumor itself which then have distance effects throughout the body, or as a result of antibodies directed against the tumor cells that cross react with other tissues.
- Signs of a PNS may precede signs of the tumor itself by weeks to months.

- The clinical signs or hematological/biochemical changes are not pathognomonic for a specific type of tumor; as PNSs are rare, these signs will typically occur with greater frequency in non-neoplastic conditions.
- Multiple PNS may be diagnosed in the same horse.
- A specific PNS is not always associated with a specific tumor type.
- Treatment of the PNS may be successful in the short term, but long-term resolution requires successful treatment of the cancer itself.
- While relatively rarely reported in horses in comparison to humans and small animals, it is possible that this is due to under recognition of PNS.

DISCLOSURE

The author has no conflicts to disclose.

REFERENCES

1. Axiak S, Johnson PJ. Paraneoplastic manifestations of cancer in horses. Equine Vet Educ 2012;24:367–76.
2. Knottenbelt DC, Patterson-Kane JC, Snalune KL. Paraneoplastic syndromes. In: Knottenbelt DC, Patterson-Kane JC, Snalune KL, editors. Equine clinical oncology. Elselvier; 2015. p. 70–84.
3. Curran K. Paraneoplastic syndromes in dogs and cats, In: *Proceedings of the ACVIM annual forum*, Phoenix, Arizona, 2019.
4. Pelosof LC, Gerber DE. Paraneoplastic syndromes: an approach to diagnosis and treatment. Mayo Clin Proc 2010;85:838–54.
5. Mair TS, Taylor FGR, Pinsent PJN. Fever of unknown origin in the horse: a review of 63 cases. Equine Vet J 1989;4:260–5.
6. Pasikhova Y, Ludlow S, Baluch A. Fever in patients with cancer. Cancer Control 2017;24:193–7.
7. Yosipovitch G. Chronic pruritis: a paraneoplastic sign. Dermatol Ther 2010;23(6): 590–6.
8. Finley MR, Rebhun WC, Dee A, et al. Paraneoplastic pruritus and alopecia in a horse with diffuse lymphoma. J Am Vet Med Assoc 1998;213:102–4.
9. Ogilvie GK. Paraneoplastic syndromes. Vet Clin North Am Equine Pract 1998;14: 439–49.
10. Taylor SD, Haldorson GJ, Vaughan B, et al. Gastric neoplasia in horses. J Vet Intern Med 2009;23:1097–102.
11. East LM, Savage CJ, Traub-Dargatz JL. Weight loss in the horse: a focus on abdominal neoplasia Equine vet. Educ Next 1999;11:174–8.
12. Nishikawa H, Goto M, Fukunishi S, et al. Cancer cachexia: its mechanism and clinical significance. Int J Mol Sci 2021;22:8491.
13. Spanton JA, Smith LJ, Sherlock SE, et al. Intestinal neoplasia: a review of 34 cases. Equine Vet Educ 2020;32:155–65.
14. Taylor SD, Pusterla N, Vaughan B, et al. Intestinal neoplasia in horses. J Vet Intern Med 2006;20:1429–36.
15. Mair TS, Rush BR, Tucker RL. Clinical and diagnostic features of thoracic neoplasia in the horse. Equine Vet Educ 2004;16:30–6.
16. Mair TS, Hillyer MH. Clinical features of lymphosarcoma in the horse: 77 cases. Equine Vet Educ 1992;4:108–13.

17. Mair TS, Brown PJ. Clinical and pathological features of thoracic neoplasia in the horse. Equine Vet J 1993;25:220–3.

18. Toussant E, Bahel-Ball E, Vekemans M, et al. Causes of fever in cancer patients (prospective study over 477 episodes). Support Care Cancer 2006;14:763–9.

19. Karcher LF, Le Net J-L, Turner BF, et al. Pseudohyperparathyroidism in a mare associated with squamous cell carcinoma of the vulva. Cornell Vet 1990;80: 153–62.

20. Meuten DJ, Price SM, Seiler RM, et al. Gastric carcinoma with pseudohyperparathyroidism in a horse. Cornell Vet 1978;68(2):179–95.

21. Esplin DG, Taylor JL. Hypercalcemia in a horse with lymphosarcoma. J Am Vet Med Assoc 1977;170:180–2.

22. Mair TS, Yeo SP, Lucke VM. Hypercalcaemia and soft tissue mineralisation associated with lymphosarcoma in two horses. Vet Rec 1990;126:99–101.

23. Cook G, Divers TJ, Rowland PH. Hypercalcaemia and erythrocytosis in a mare associated with a metastatic carcinoma. Equine Vet J 1995;27:316–8.

24. Fix AS, Miller LD. Equine adrenocortical carcinoma with hypercalcemia. Vet Pathol 1987;24:190–2.

25. Rosol TJ, Nagode LA, Robertson JT, et al. Humoral hypercalcemia of malignancy associated with ameloblastoma in a horse. J Am Vet Med Assoc 1994;204: 1930–3.

26. Edwards DF, Parker JW, Wilkinson JE, et al. Plasma cell myeloma in the horse. a case report and literature review. J Vet Intern Med 1993;7:169–76.

27. Pusterla N, Stacy BA, Vernau W, et al. Immunoglobulin A monoclonal gammopathy in two horses with multiple myeloma. Vet Rec 2004;155:19–23.

28. Barton MH, Sharma P, LeRoy BE, et al. Hypercalcemia and high serum parathyroid hormone-related protein concentration in a horse with multiple myeloma. J Am Vet Med Assoc 2004;225:409–13.

29. Darby S, Porter E, Beatty SSK, et al. Primary hyperparathyroidism in a quarter horse mare associated with a chief cell adenoma. J Equine Vet Sci 2020;95: 103302.

30. LeRoy B, Woolums A, Wass J, et al. The relationship between serum calcium concentration and outcome in horses with renal failure presented to referral hospitals. J Vet Intern Med 2011;25:1426–30.

31. Gorenberg EB, Johnson AL, Magdesian KG, et al. Diagnosis and treatment of confirmed and suspected primary hyperparathyroidism in equids: 17 cases (1999-2016). Equine Vet J 2020;52:83–90.

32. Grubb TL, Foreman JH, Benson GJ, et al. Hemodynamic effects of calcium gluconate administered to conscious horses. J vet int Med 1996;10:401–4.

33. Van de Kolk JH. Humeral hypercalcaemia of malignancy or pseudohyperparathyroidism in the horse. Equine Vet Educ 2007;19:384–6.

34. Tonon CR, Silva TAAL, Pereira FWL, et al. A review of current concepts in the pathophysiology, etiology, diagnosis and management of hypercalcemia. Med Sci Monit 2022;28:e935821.

35. Atkins CE. Cardiac manifestations of systemic and metabolic disease. In: Fox PR, Sisson D, Moïse NS, editors. Textbook of canine and feline cardiology. 2nd edn. Pennsylvania: W.B. Saunders; 1999. p. 768–70.

36. Reef VB. Arrhythmias. In: Marr CM, editor. Cardiology of the horse. 1st edn. London: W.B. Saunders; 1999. p. 204–7.

37. Mair TS, Tucker RL. Hypertrophic osteopathy (Marie's disease) in horses. Equine Vet Educ 2004;16(6):308–11.

38. Mair TS, Dyson SJ, Fraser JA, et al. Hypertrophic osteopathy (Marie's disease) in equidae: a review of twenty-four cases. Equine Vet J 1996;28:256–62.
39. van der Kolk JH, Geelen SN, Jonker FH, et al. Hypertrophic osteopathy associated with ovarian carcinoma in a mare. Vet Rec 1998;143:172–3.
40. Schleining JA, Voss ED. Hypertrophic osteopathy secondary to gastric squamous cell carcinoma in a horse. Equine Vet Educ 2004;16:304–7.
41. Alexander JE, Keown GH, Palotay JL. Granular cell myoblastoma with hypertrophic pulmonary osteoarthropathy in a mare. J Am Vet Med Assoc 1965;146: 703–8.
42. Sutton RH, Coleman GT. A pulmonary granular cell tumour with associated hypertrophic osteopathy in a horse. N Z Vet J 1995;43:123.
43. Heinola T, Heikkila M, Ruohoniemi M, et al. Hypertrophic pulmonary osteopathy associated with granular cell tumor in a mare. Vet Rec 2001;149:307–8.
44. Tomlinson JE, Divers TJ, McDonough SP, et al. Hypertrophic osteopathy secondary to nodular pulmonary fibrosis in a horse. J Vet Intern Med 2011;25:153–7.
45. Lavoie J-P, Carlson GP, George L. Hypertrophic osteopathy in three horses and a pony. J Am Vet Med Assoc 1992;201:1900–4.
46. Chakraborty RK, Sharma S. Secondary hypertrophic osteoarthropathy. In: StatPearls [Internet]. Treasure Island (FL): StatPearls Publishing; 2023.
47. Lenehan TM, Fetter AW. Hypertrophic osteopathy. In: Newton CD, Nunamaker CM, editors. Textbook of small animal orthopaedics. Philadelphia: J B Lippincott Company; 1985. p. 603–9.
48. Dickinson CJ, Martin JF. Megakaryocytes and platelet clumps as the cause of finger clubbing. Lancet 1987;2:1434–5.
49. Yao Q, Altman RD, Brahn E. Periostitis and hypertrophic pulmonary osteoarthropathy: report of 2 cases and review of the literature. Semin Arthritis Rheum 2009; 38:458–66.
50. Martinez-Lavin M. Exploring the cause of the most ancient clinical sign of medicine: finger clubbing. Semin Arthritis Rheum 2007;36:380–5.
51. Martinez-Lavin M, Vargas A, Rivera-Viñas M. Hypertrophic osteoarthropathy: a palindrome with a pathogenic connotation. Curr Opin Rheumatol 2008;20:88–91.
52. Atkinson S, Fox SB. Vascular endothelial growth factor (VEGF)-A and platelet-derived growth factor (PDGF) play a central role in the pathogenesis of digital clubbing. J Pathol 2004;203:721–8.
53. Silveira L, Martínez-Lavín M, Pineda C, et al. Vascular endothelial growth factor in hypertrophic osteoarthropathy. Clin Exp Rheumatol 2000;18:57–62.
54. Flavell G. Reversal of pulmonary hypertrophic osteoarthropathy by vagotomy. Lancet 1956;270:260–2.
55. Bazar KA, Yun AJ, Lee PY. Hypertrophic osteoarthropathy may be a marker of underlying sympathetic bias. Med Hypotheses 2004;63:357–61.
56. Chaffin MK, Ruoff WW, Schmitz DG, et al. Regression of hypertrophic osteopathy in a filly following successful management of an intrathoracic abscess. Equine Vet J 1990;22:62–5.
57. Munoz A, Riber C, Satue K, et al. Multiple myeloma in horses, dogs and cats: a comparative review focussed on clinical signs and pathogenesis. In: Hajek R, editor. Multiple myeloma - a quick reflection on the fast progress. InTech; 2013. p. 289–326.
58. Badial PR, Tallmadge RL, Miller A, et al. Applied protein and molecular techniques for characterization of B cell neoplasms in horses. Clin Vaccine Immunol 2015;22:1133–45.

59. Munoz A, Riber C, Trigo P, et al. Hematopoietic neoplasias in horses: myeloproliferative and lymphoproliferative disorders. J Equine Sci 2009;20(4):59–72.
60. Meyer J, DeLay J, Bienzle D. Clinical, laboratory and histopathologic features of equine lymphoma. Vet Pathol 2006;43:914–24.
61. Hayes AM, Kastl B, Perry E, et al. Multiple myeloma presenting as blepharitis in a horse. Vet Clin Pathol 2023;52:514–20.
62. Kent JE, Roberts CA. Serum protein changes in four horses with monoclonal gammopathy. Equine Vet J 1990;22:373–6.
63. Jacobs RM, Kociba GJ, Ruoff WW. Monoclonal gammopathy in a horse with defective hemostasis. Vet Pathol 1983;20:643–7.
64. Eberhardt CE, Malbon A, Rion B, et al. K Light-chain monoclonal gammopathy and cast nephropathy in a horse with multiple myeloma. J Am Vet Med Assoc 2018;253:1177–83.
65. Morton AJ, Davis JL, Redding WR, et al. Nonsecretory multiple myeloma in a horse. Equine Vet Educ 2007;19:564–8.
66. Markel MD, Dorr TE. Multiple myeloma in a horse. J Am Vet Med Assoc 1986;188: 621–3.
67. MacAllister C, Qualls C Jr, Tyler R, et al. Multiple myeloma in a horse. J Am Vet Med Assoc 1987;191:337–9.
68. Geelen SN, Bernardina WE, Grinwis GC, et al. Monoclonal Gammopathy in a Dutch Warmblood Mare. Vet Q 1997;19:29–32.
69. McConkey S, Lopez A, Pringle J. Extramedullary Plasmacytoma in a Horse with Ptyalism and Dysphagia. J Vet Diagn Invest 2000;12:282–4.
70. Kim DY, Taylor HW, Eades SC, et al. Systemic AL amyloidosis associated with multiple myeloma in a horse. Vet Pathol 2005;42:81–4.
71. Henry M, Prasse K, White S. Hemorrhagic diathesis caused by multiple myeloma in a thee-month-old foal. J Am Vet Med Assoc 1989;194:392–4.
72. Drew RA, Greatorex JC. Vertebral plasma cell myeloma causing posterior paralysis in a horse. Equine Vet J 1974;6:131–4.
73. Southwood LL, Schott HC, Henry CJ, et al. Disseminated hemangiosarcoma in the horse: 35 cases. J Vet Intern Med 2000;14:105–9.
74. Roby KA, Beech J, Bloom JC, et al. Hepatocellular carcinoma associated with erythrocytosis and hypoglycemia in a yearling filly. J Am Vet Med Assoc 1990;196: 465–7.
75. Lennox TJ, Wilson JH, Hayden DW, et al. Hepatoblastoma with erythrocytosis in a young female horse. J Am Vet Med Assoc 2000;216:718–21.
76. Beeler-Marfisi J, Arroyo L, Caswell JL, et al. Equine primary liver tumors: a case series and review of the literature. J Vet Diagnostic Invest 2010;22:174–83.
77. Tirosh-Levy S, Perl S, Valentine BA, et al. Erythrocytosis and fatigue fractures associated with hepatoblastoma in a 3-year-old gelding. J S Afr Vet Assoc 2019;28:90.
78. Axon JE, Russell CM, Begg AP, et al. Erythrocytosis and pleural effusion associated with a hepatoblastoma in a Thoroughbred yearling. Aust Vet J 2008;86: 329–33.
79. Gold JR, Warren AL, French TW, et al. What is your diagnosis? Biopsy impression smear of a hepatic mass in a yearling Thoroughbred filly. Vet Clin Pathol 2008;37: 339–43.
80. Koch TG, Wen X, Bienzle D. Lymphoma, erythrocytosis, and tumor erythropoietin gene expression in a horse. J Vet Intern Med 2006;20:1251–5.
81. Aleman M, Costa LRR, Crowe C, et al. Presumed neuroglycopenia caused by severe hypoglycemia in horses. J Vet Intern Med 2018;32:1731–9.

82. Baker JL, Aleman M, Madigan J. Intermittent hypoglycemia in a horse with anaplastic carcinoma of the kidney. J Am Vet Med Assoc 2001;218:235–7.
83. LaCarrubba AM, Johnson PJ, Whitney MS, et al. Hypocalcaemia and acute tumour lysis syndrome associated with peritoneal mesothelioma in a horse. J Vet Intern Med 2006;20:1018–22.
84. West HJ, Kelly DF, Ritchie HE. Renal carcinomatosis in a horse. Equine Vet J 1987;19:548–51.
85. Wong D, Hepworth K, Yaeger M, et al. Imaging diagnosis hypoglycemia associated with cholangiocarcinoma and peritoneal carcinomatosis in a horse. Vet Radiol Ultrasound 2015;56:E9–12.
86. Sakamoto T, Kaneshige H, Takeshi A, et al. Localized pleural mesothelioma with elevation of high molecular weight insulin-like growth factor II and hypoglycemia. Chest 1994;106:965–7.
87. Owen RA, Haywood S, Kelly DF. Clinical course of renal adenocarcinoma associated with hypercupraemia in a horse. Vet Rec 1986;119:291–4.
88. Williams MA, Dowling PM, Angarano DW, et al. Paraneoplastic bullous stomatitis in a horse. J Am Vet Med Assoc 1995;207:331–4.
89. Onyema MC, Drakou EE, Dimitriadis GK. Endocrine abnormality in paraneoplastic syndrome. Best Pract Res Clin Endocrinol Metabol 2022;36:101621.
90. Abbott B, Stephenson R, Fox RI. Concurrent granulomatous dermatitis and malignant granulosa cell tumour in a mare. Equine Vet Educ 2004;16:255–60.
91. Linke RP, Geisel O, Mann K, et al. Equine cutaneous amyloidosis derived from an immunoglobulin lambda-light chain. Immunohistochemical, immunochemical and chemical results. Biol Chem Hoppe Seyler 1991;372:835–43.
92. Van Andel AC, Gruys E, Kroneman J, et al. Amyloid in the horse: a report of nine cases. Equine Vet J 1998;20:277–85.
93. Gilligan M, McGuigan C, McKeon A. Paraneoplastic neurologic disorders. Curr Neurol Neurosci Rep 2023;23:67–82.
94. Gliatto JM, Alroy J, Gliatto JM, et al. Cutaneous amyloidosis in a horse with lymphoma. Vet Rec 1995;137:68–9.

Moving?

Make sure your subscription moves with you!

To notify us of your new address, find your **Clinics Account Number** (located on your mailing label above your name), and contact customer service at:

Email: journalscustomerservice-usa@elsevier.com

800-654-2452 (subscribers in the U.S. & Canada)
314-447-8871 (subscribers outside of the U.S. & Canada)

Fax number: 314-447-8029

Elsevier Health Sciences Division
Subscription Customer Service
3251 Riverport Lane
Maryland Heights, MO 63043

*To ensure uninterrupted delivery of your subscription, please notify us at least 4 weeks in advance of move.

Printed and bound by CPI Group (UK) Ltd, Croydon, CR0 4YY

08/05/2025

01864724-0002